Chair Yoga For Seniors Over 70

A Comprehensive 8-Week Guide to Senior Health and Fitness through Stretching

Daniel Moore

Table of Content

Copyright Page

Disclaimer

Before embarking on any new exercise program, including chair yoga, it is essential to consult with a healthcare provider, especially for individuals with pre-existing health conditions or concerns. This book is intended to complement, not replace, professional medical advice and treatment

PREFACE

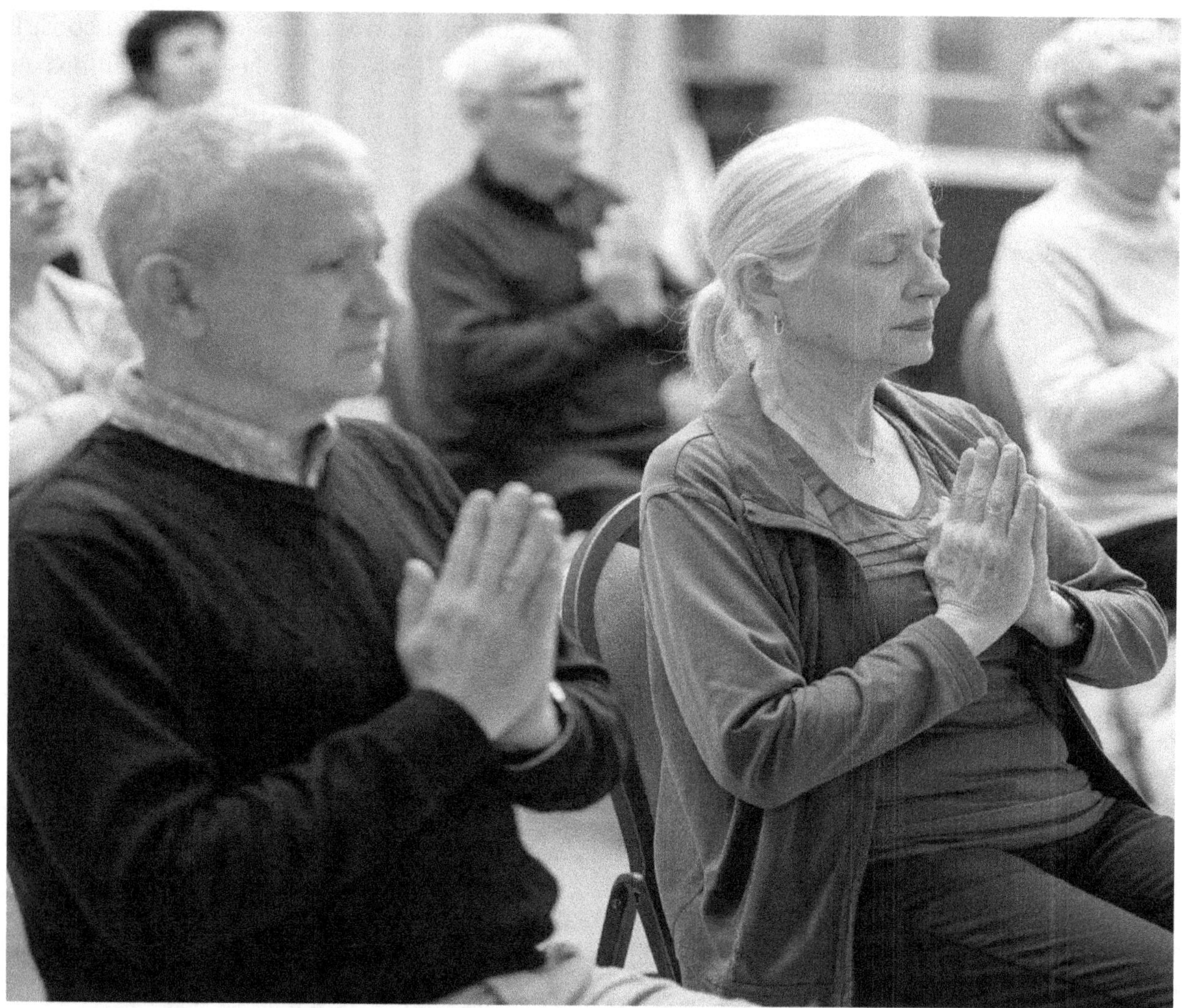

When I reflect on my journey as a professional trainer specializing in chair yoga for seniors, I am filled with a profound sense of gratitude and fulfillment. My name is Joshua Isaac, and for over two decades, I have dedicated my life to enhancing the health and well-being of seniors through the gentle practice of chair yoga. This book, Chair Yoga for Seniors Over 70, is the culmination of years of experience, passion, and unwavering commitment to making fitness accessible and enjoyable for our beloved elders.

Growing up in the vibrant and diverse city of San Francisco, I was fortunate to be surrounded by a community that valued health, wellness, and the importance of staying active at every age. However, amidst the hustle and bustle of urban life, I witnessed a growing concern among my grandparents and their peers. They grappled with the challenges of maintaining their physical health, battling the effects of aging that often led to discomfort, reduced mobility, and a sense of isolation. Their struggles ignited a spark within me—a desire to make a tangible difference in their lives.

My interest in fitness began early. As a child, I watched my grandparents navigate their daily routines with grace and resilience, despite the physical limitations that came with age. Their determination to stay active, even when faced with pain and stiffness, was both inspiring and heart-wrenching. I saw firsthand how regular physical activity could transform their days, bringing moments of joy, relief, and a renewed sense of independence. However, I also saw the barriers they faced—whether it was the intimidation of traditional exercise classes, the fear of injury, or simply not knowing where to start.

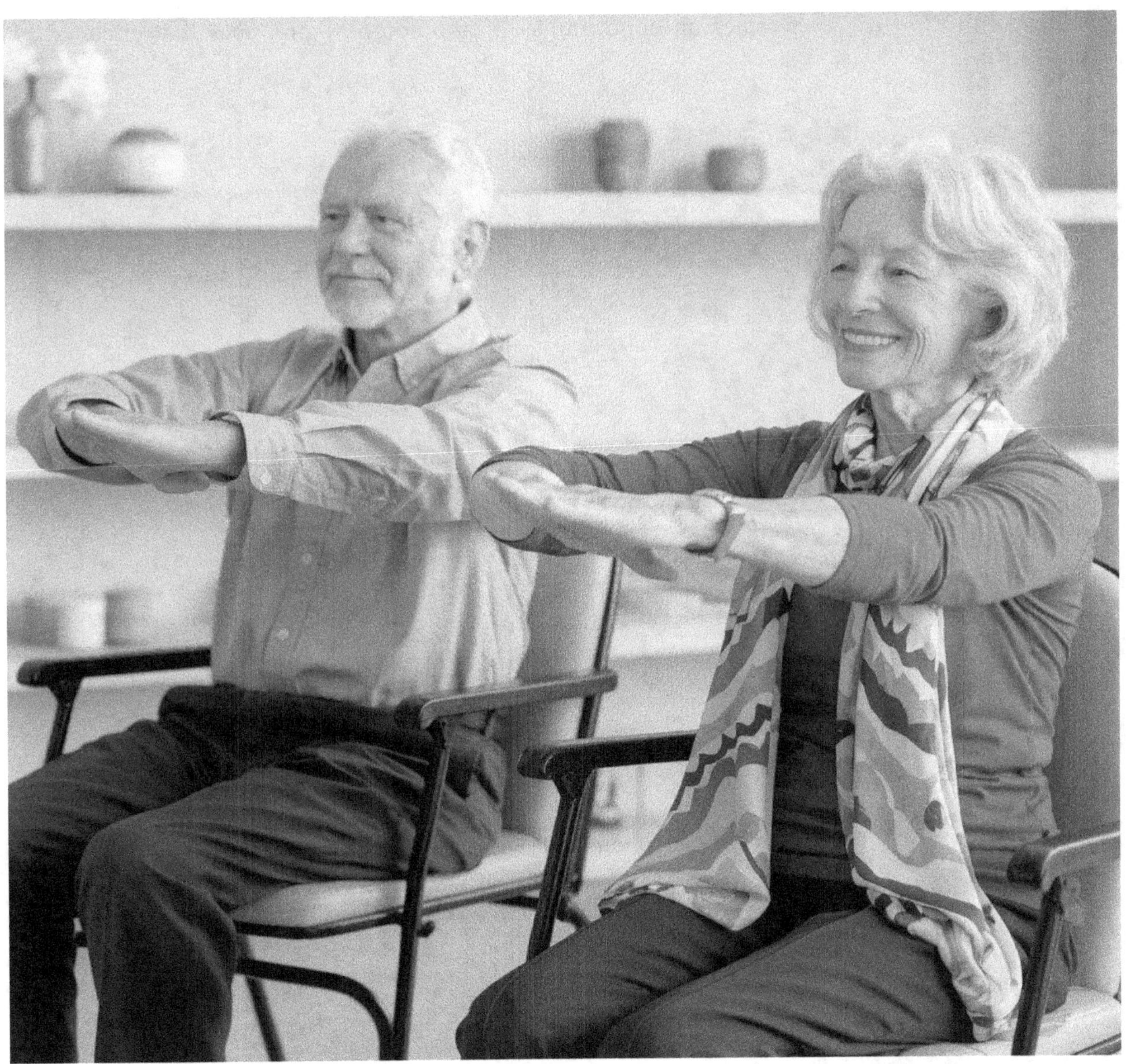

These observations led me to pursue a career in fitness with a focus on senior health. I enrolled in a specialized program in chair yoga, a practice that combines the principles of traditional yoga with modifications to accommodate those with limited mobility. Chair yoga became my passion, as it offered a safe, effective, and accessible way for seniors to improve their strength, flexibility, and overall well-being without the stress and strain often associated with other forms of exercise.

Over the years, I have had the privilege of working with countless seniors, each with their unique stories and challenges. From helping a widow regain her confidence after a hip replacement to assisting a retired teacher in overcoming chronic back pain, these experiences have been both humbling and rewarding. Each session, each success story, has reinforced my belief in the transformative power of chair yoga. It has shown me that age is not a barrier to maintaining an active and fulfilling life, but rather an opportunity to embrace new practices that enhance our quality of life.

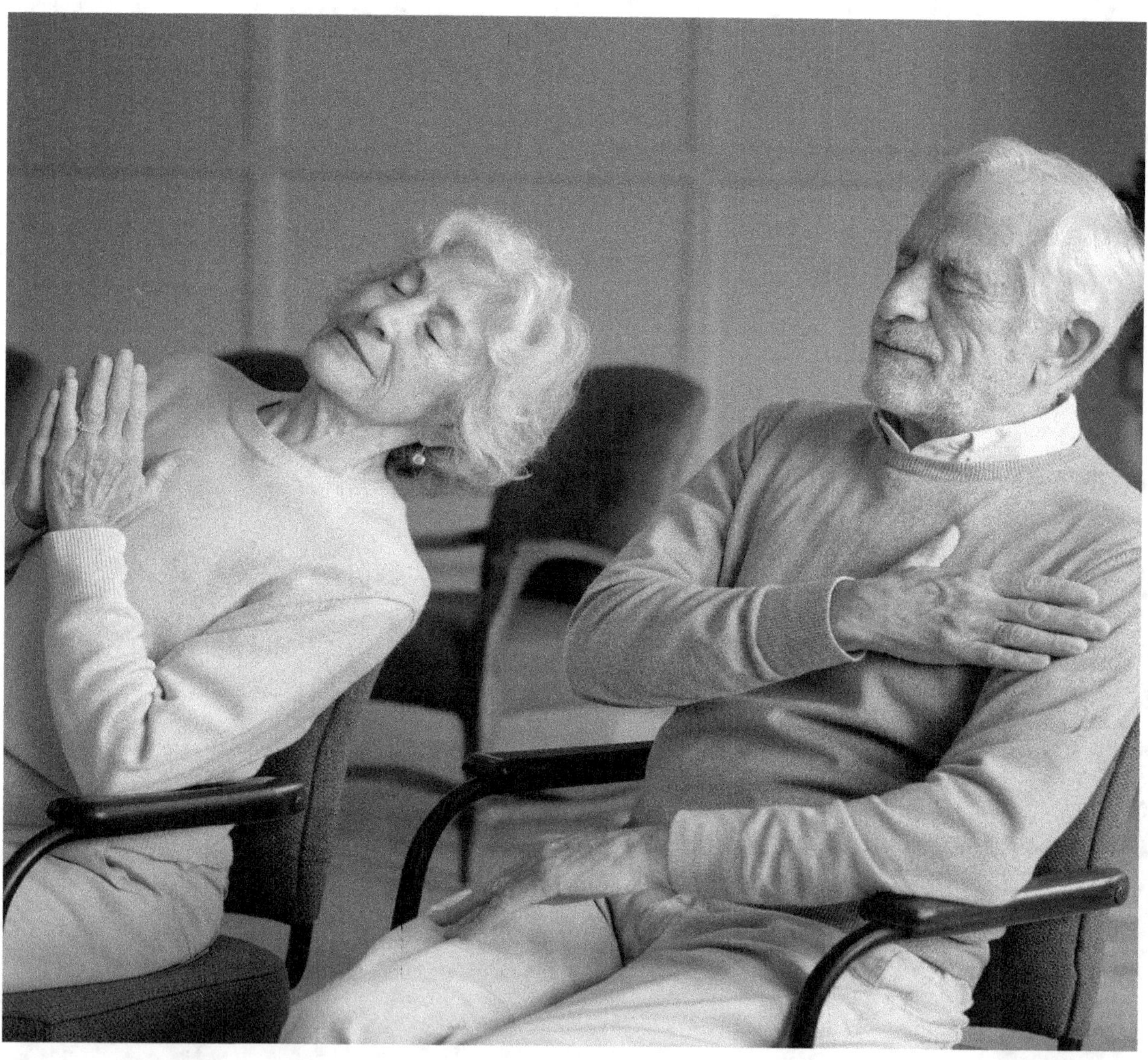

One of the most poignant moments in my career came when I began conducting classes at a local senior center. I remember meeting Eleanor, an 82-year-old woman who had recently lost her husband. She was hesitant to join the class, unsure if she could keep up with the exercises. Over time, Eleanor not only regained her physical strength but also found solace and a sense of community through our sessions. Her laughter, stories, and gradual transformation were a testament to the profound impact of chair yoga on both body and spirit.

This book is a reflection of those experiences and the lessons I have learned along the way. Chair Yoga for Seniors Over 70 is designed to be more than just a collection of exercises; it is a comprehensive guide that addresses the unique needs of seniors, offering them a pathway to improved health, enhanced mobility, and a better quality of life. Whether you are a senior yourself, a caregiver, or a fitness professional looking to expand your repertoire, this book provides practical, easy-to-follow instructions and insights that can make a meaningful difference.

In crafting this guide, I drew upon the principles that have guided my practice for years. Safety and comfort are paramount, and every exercise is tailored to accommodate varying levels of mobility and fitness. The routines are structured to build strength gradually, improve flexibility, and promote mental well-being through mindful breathing and relaxation techniques. Each chapter delves into different aspects of senior health, from managing arthritis and alleviating chronic pain to enhancing joint mobility and integrating yoga into daily life.

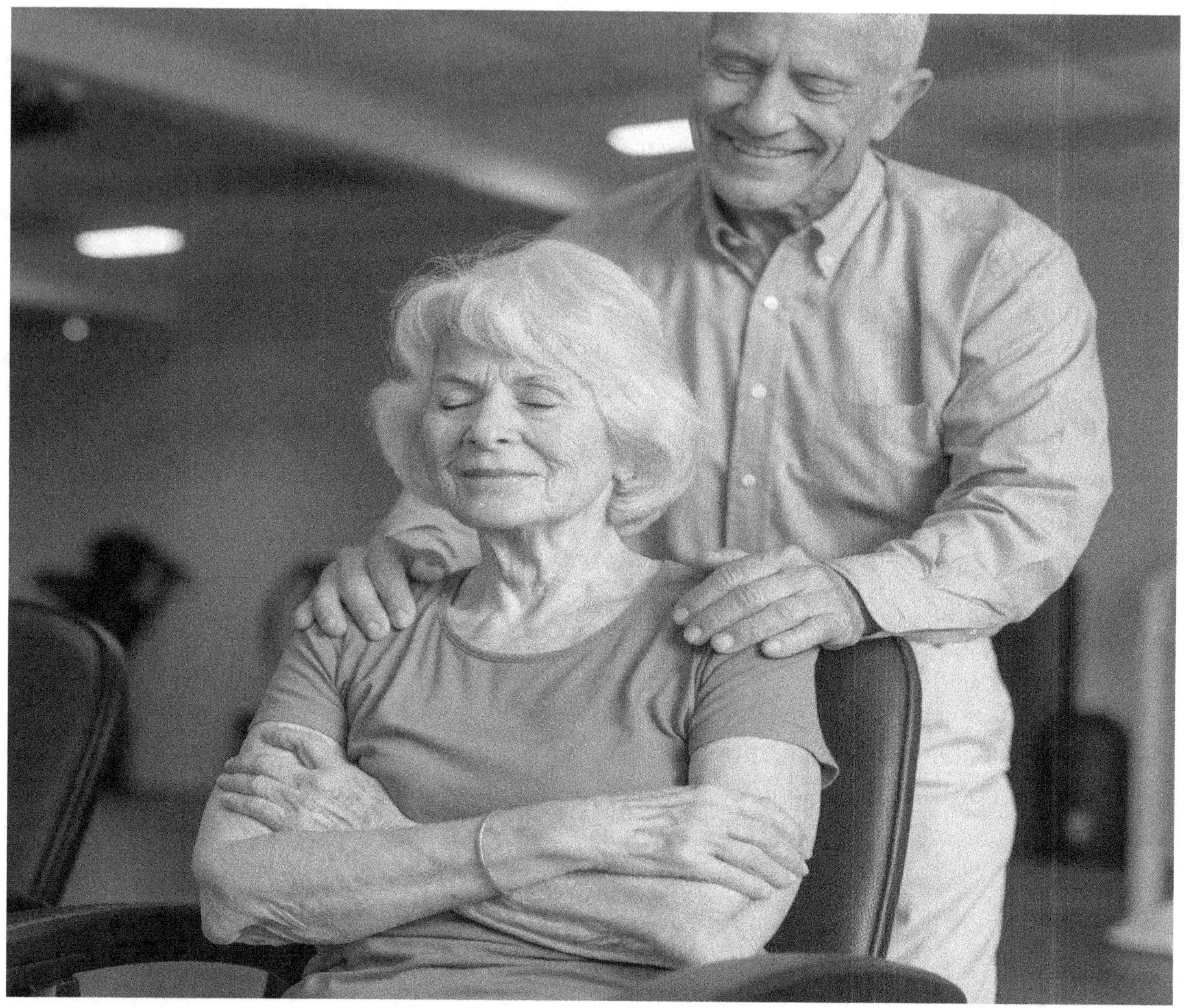

One of the key elements I emphasize in this book is the importance of consistency. Just as with any form of exercise, the benefits of chair yoga are most pronounced when practiced regularly. I have seen seniors transform their lives by committing to a routine, experiencing not only physical improvements but also enhanced mental clarity and emotional resilience. This guide provides a structured 8-week program, breaking down each week's focus to ensure a balanced and effective approach to fitness that is both sustainable and rewarding.

Another cornerstone of this book is the holistic approach to health. Chair yoga is not just about physical movement; it encompasses mental and emotional well-being as well. Through guided stretches, strengthening exercises, and mindfulness practices, seniors can achieve a harmonious balance that supports overall health. I have incorporated elements such as meditation, breathing exercises, and posture improvement techniques to provide a comprehensive wellness plan that addresses the multifaceted nature of aging.

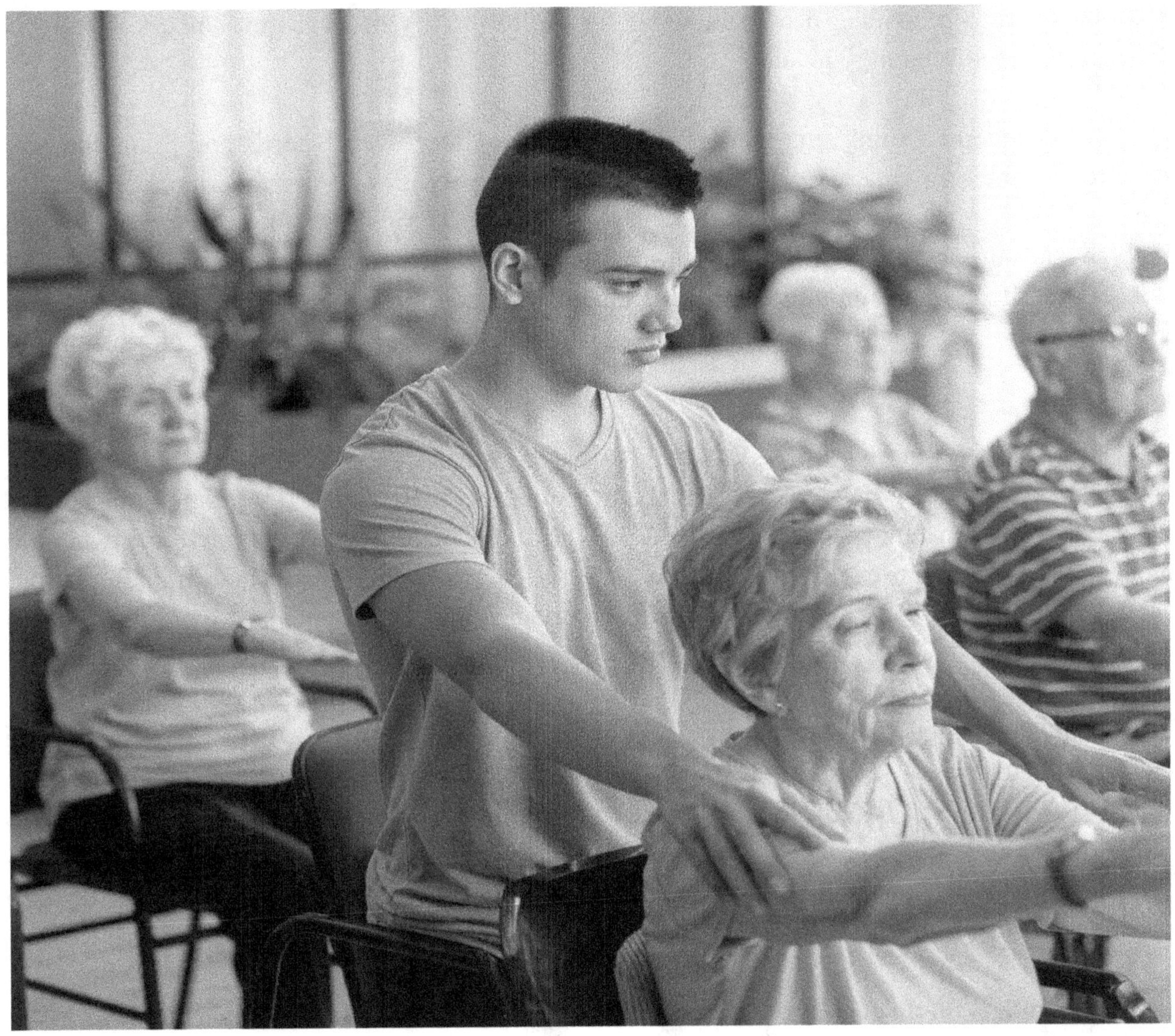

Throughout my career, I have also witnessed the incredible sense of community that chair yoga fosters. Seniors often form strong bonds with their peers during classes, sharing their journeys, challenges, and triumphs. This sense of camaraderie not only enhances the exercise experience but also combats feelings of loneliness and isolation that can accompany aging. In this book, I include tips and strategies for creating a supportive and engaging environment, whether in a group class setting or in the comfort of one's own home.

In addition to the physical and mental benefits, chair yoga offers practical advantages that make it an ideal choice for seniors. The seated position reduces the risk of falls and injuries, making it a safer option compared to traditional yoga practices. The exercises can be performed anywhere, without the need for specialized equipment or a large space, making it accessible for those with limited mobility or who prefer to exercise in familiar surroundings. Moreover, chair yoga can be easily adapted to individual needs, allowing seniors to modify movements as necessary to suit their comfort and capability levels.

As I embarked on writing this book, I was mindful of the diverse needs and preferences of seniors. I wanted to create a guide that is inclusive, respectful, and empowering, encouraging seniors to take charge of their health in a way that feels right for them. Each exercise is accompanied by detailed instructions, illustrations, and tips to ensure that it can be performed safely and effectively. Additionally, I have included personal anecdotes and success stories to inspire and motivate readers, highlighting the real-life impact of chair yoga on senior health and happiness.

One of the most rewarding aspects of my work has been seeing the profound changes that chair yoga can bring about. Seniors who once felt limited by their physical conditions often find renewed vitality and independence through regular practice. They report improvements in their mobility, reduced pain levels, and a greater sense of overall well-being. These transformations extend beyond the physical, fostering a positive mindset and a resilient spirit that helps seniors navigate the challenges of aging with grace and confidence.

In writing Chair Yoga for Seniors Over 70, my goal is to share the knowledge and insights I have gained over the years, providing a valuable resource that can help seniors live healthier, more active lives. I have structured the book to be user-friendly, with clear instructions and progressive routines that build upon each other to ensure continuous improvement. The 8-week plan is designed to guide readers through a journey of discovery and growth, allowing them to experience the full spectrum of benefits that chair yoga has to offer.

I am particularly proud of the sections that address specific health concerns such as arthritis, chronic pain, and joint mobility. These are common issues that can significantly impact a senior's quality of life, and chair yoga offers a natural, non-invasive way to manage and alleviate these conditions. By focusing on gentle movements and targeted exercises, this guide provides practical solutions that can help seniors regain control over their health and enjoy a more active, fulfilling life.

Furthermore, the integration of yoga into daily life is a theme that runs throughout the book. I believe that yoga should not be confined to the exercise session but should be a seamless part of one's everyday routine. The strategies and tips I provide are aimed at helping seniors incorporate yoga into their daily activities, making it a sustainable and integral part of their lifestyle. This holistic approach ensures that the benefits of yoga extend beyond the mat, enhancing overall well-being and promoting a balanced, harmonious life.

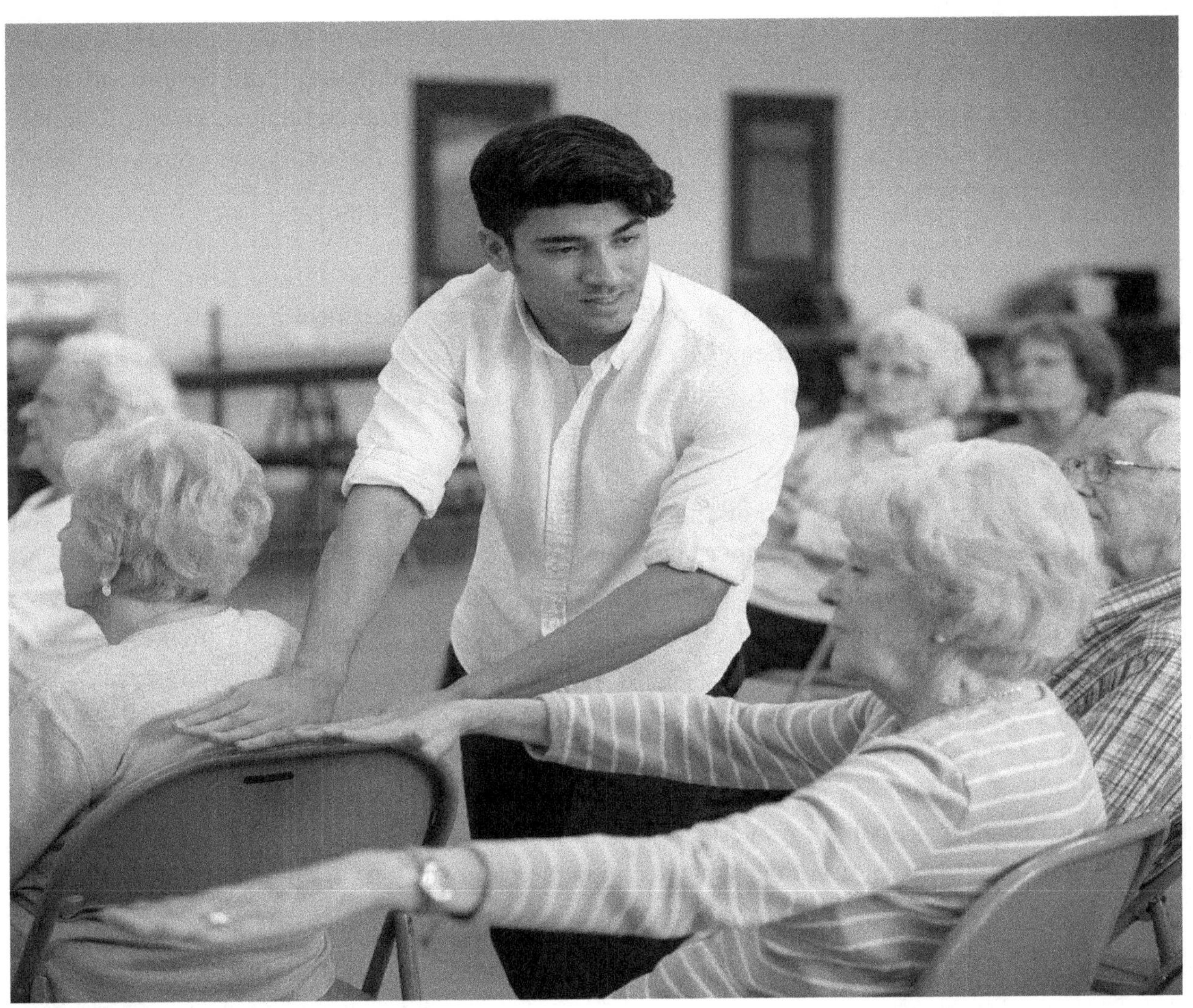

As I look back on my journey, I am reminded of the countless lives that have been touched and transformed through chair yoga. Each senior I have worked with has taught me something valuable, reinforcing the importance of patience, compassion, and adaptability in my practice. Their stories of perseverance and triumph are a constant source of inspiration, driving me to continue expanding my knowledge and refining my methods to better serve the senior community.

This book is my way of giving back to the community that has given me so much. It is a labor of love, born out of a deep-seated desire to make a positive impact on the lives of seniors. I have poured my heart and soul into every page, ensuring that it is not only informative but also engaging and empowering. My hope is that Chair Yoga for Seniors Over 70 will become a trusted companion for seniors on their journey to better health, providing them with the tools and confidence they need to embrace a more active and vibrant life.

In the pages that follow, you will find a wealth of knowledge and practical advice designed to guide you through the practice of chair yoga. From foundational exercises to advanced techniques, each section is crafted to address the unique needs and challenges faced by seniors. The routines are carefully structured to build strength, enhance flexibility, and promote mental clarity, ensuring a comprehensive approach to health and wellness.

I encourage you to approach this book with an open mind and a willing heart. Embrace the practice of chair yoga as a means to not only improve your physical health but also to cultivate a deeper sense of peace and well-being. Remember that every journey begins with a single step, and by committing to this practice, you are taking a significant step towards a healthier, more fulfilling life.

As you embark on this journey, know that you are not alone. The senior community is a vibrant and supportive network, and together, we can achieve remarkable things. Whether you are seeking to alleviate pain, improve mobility, or simply enhance your overall health, chair yoga offers a path that is both gentle and effective. This book is your guide, your mentor, and your companion as you navigate the beautiful journey of aging with grace, strength, and vitality.

In closing, I would like to extend my deepest gratitude to the seniors who have entrusted me with their health and wellness over the years. Your resilience, courage, and unwavering spirit have been the driving force behind my work. It is your stories, your successes, and your unwavering commitment to staying active that have inspired me to create this book. May Chair Yoga for Seniors Over 70 be a beacon of hope, a source of strength, and a testament to the incredible potential that lies within each of us, regardless of age.

Thank you for allowing me to be a part of your journey. Together, let us embrace the transformative power of chair yoga and celebrate the beauty of aging with health, happiness, and grace.

Daniel Moore

Chapter 1

INTRODUCTION TO CHAIR YOGA

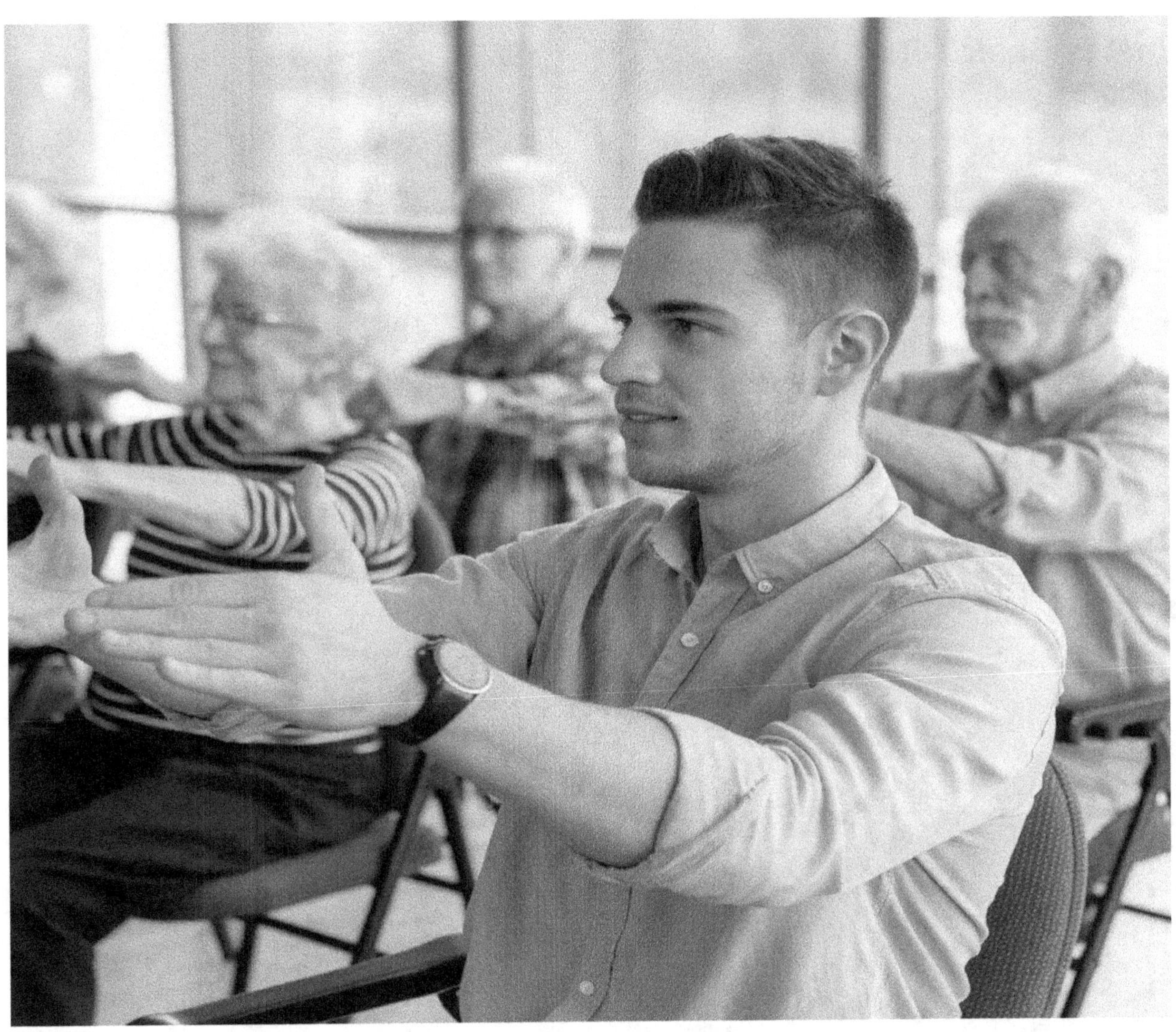

Welcome to the transformative world of Chair Yoga, a specially designed practice that brings the benefits of traditional yoga to seniors over 70 in a safe, accessible, and comfortable manner. In this introductory chapter, I'll explore the fundamental principles of Chair Yoga, highlighting its unique ability to enhance physical health, mental well-being, and overall quality of life without the need for standing or extensive flexibility. You will discover how Chair Yoga accommodates varying mobility levels, making it an ideal exercise regimen for those with limited movement or chronic conditions. I delve into the numerous advantages of incorporating Chair Yoga into your daily routine, including improved joint health, increased flexibility, reduced pain, and enhanced relaxation. Additionally, this chapter provides an overview of the essential equipment and space setup, ensuring that you can practice confidently and effectively at home or in a community setting. Whether you are new to yoga or seeking a gentle yet effective way to stay active, this introduction sets the stage for a rewarding journey towards greater strength, balance, and serenity through Chair Yoga.

What is Chair Yoga?

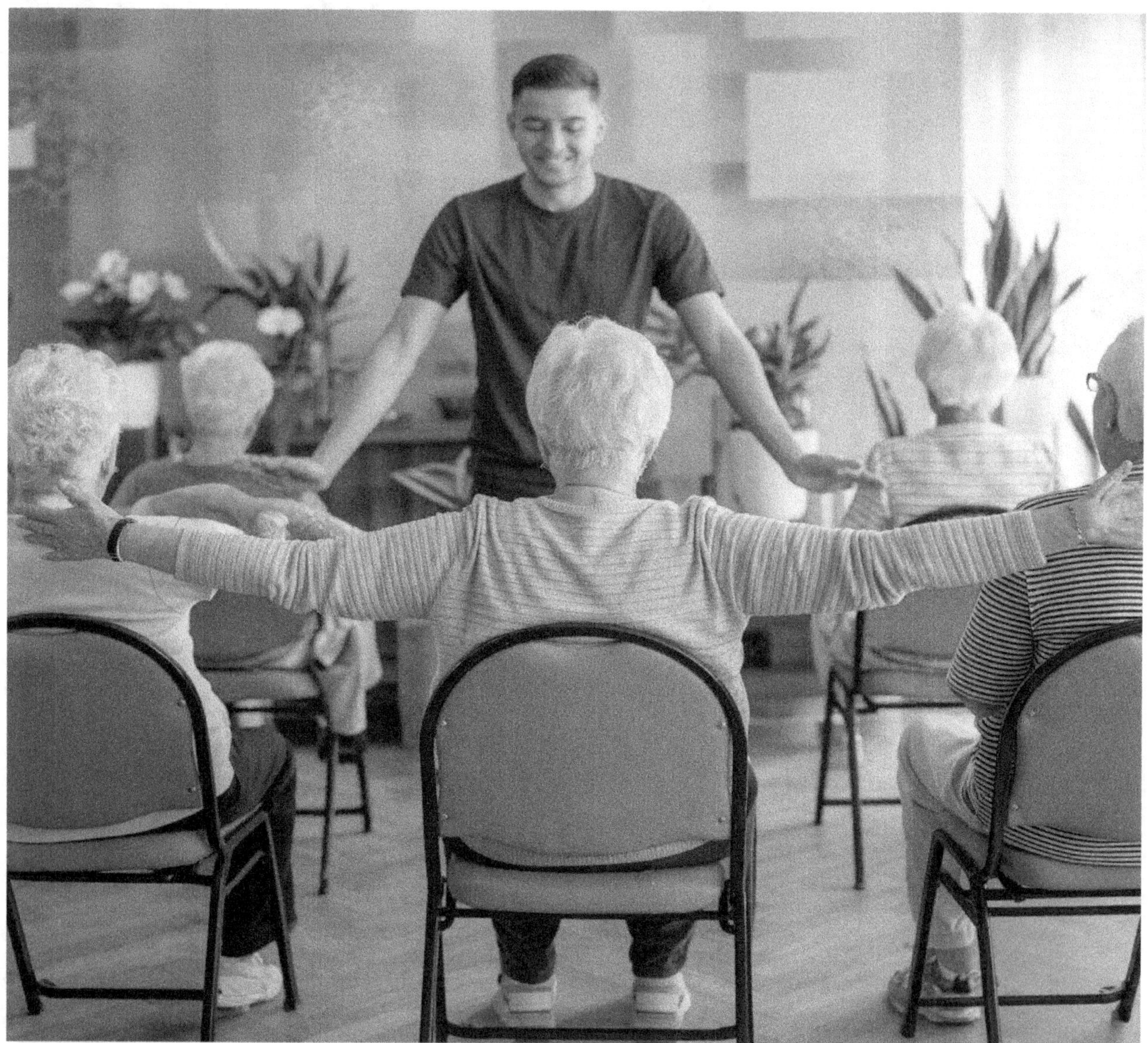

Definition and Overview

Chair Yoga is a gentle form of yoga that is practiced while sitting on a chair or using a chair for support. It is specifically designed to make yoga accessible to individuals who may have limited mobility, balance issues, or other physical constraints that make traditional yoga poses challenging. By adapting the traditional yoga poses to a seated or supported position, Chair Yoga allows seniors over 70 to enjoy the numerous benefits of yoga without the need to stand or kneel.

At its core, Chair Yoga emphasizes the same principles as traditional yoga, including breath control, meditation, and the flow of movement. However, it modifies the intensity and complexity of poses to accommodate the needs of older adults. This approach ensures that seniors can engage in physical activity safely and comfortably, enhancing their overall well-being without the risk of injury.

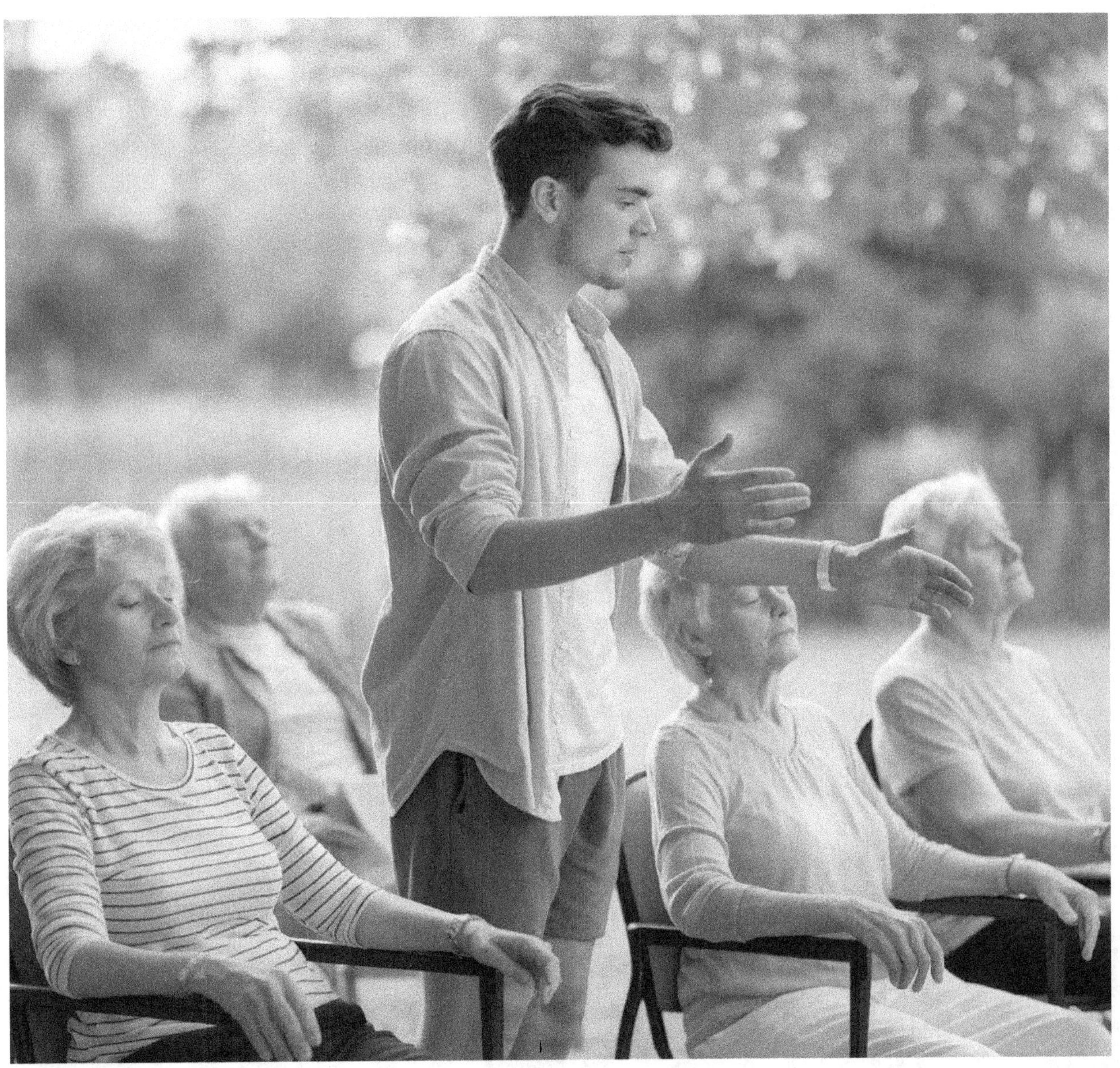

Chair Yoga incorporates a variety of movements that target different areas of the body, promoting flexibility, strength, and balance. These movements are often slower and more controlled, allowing practitioners to focus on proper alignment and mindful breathing. The seated nature of Chair Yoga also makes it easier to maintain stability, making it an ideal practice for those who may struggle with balance or fear falling.

One of the key advantages of Chair Yoga is its adaptability. Whether you are confined to a wheelchair or have the ability to stand with assistance, Chair Yoga can be tailored to fit your specific needs. This flexibility ensures that everyone, regardless of their physical condition, can participate and reap the benefits of yoga. Additionally, Chair Yoga can be practiced in various settings, including at home, in community centers, or even in office environments.

Overall, Chair Yoga serves as a bridge between traditional yoga and the unique requirements of seniors. It provides a holistic approach to health and wellness, addressing both physical and mental aspects. By incorporating Chair Yoga into their routine, seniors can improve their quality of life, maintain independence, and enjoy a greater sense of vitality and peace.

History and Evolution

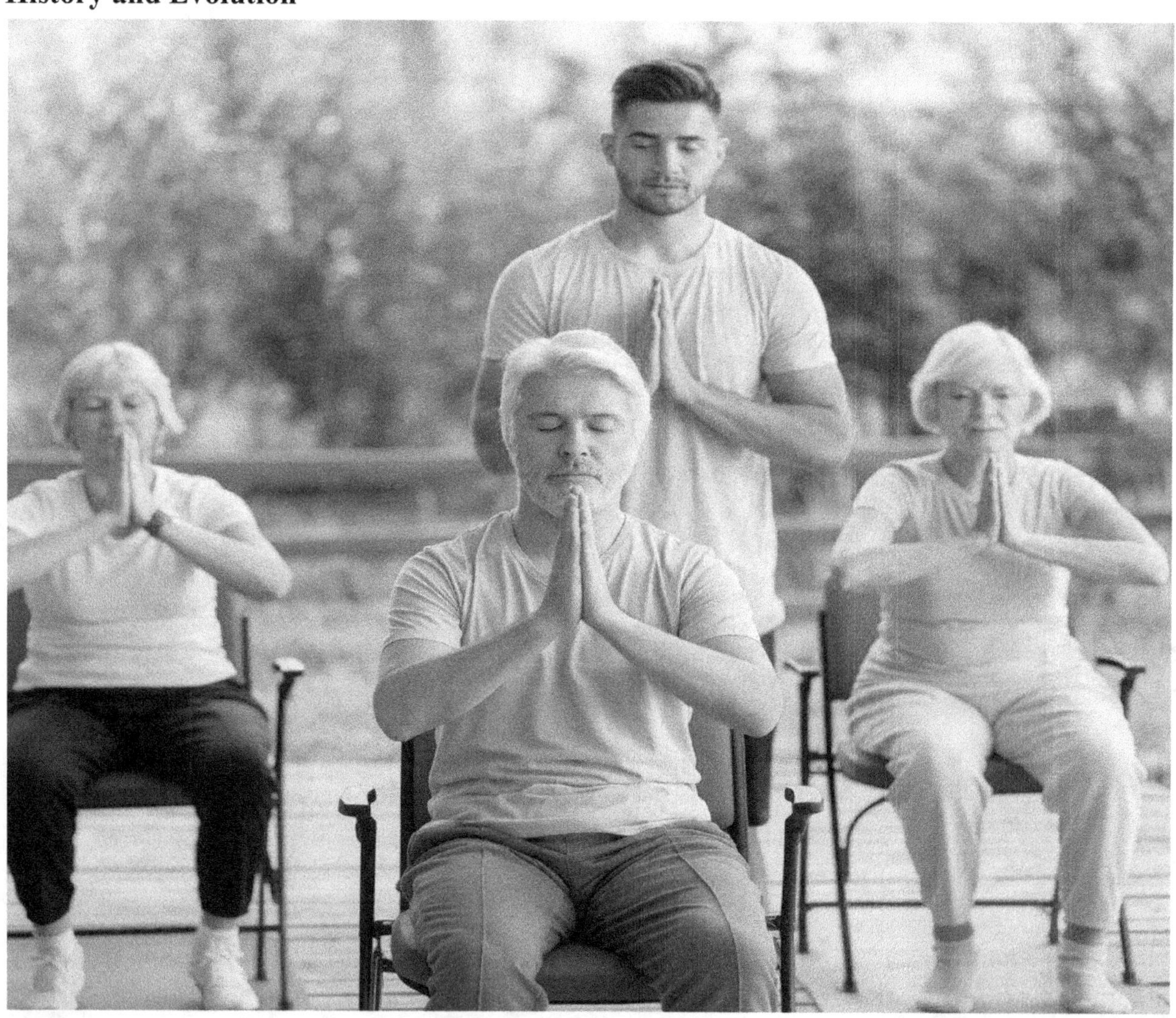

The concept of Chair Yoga emerged as a response to the growing need for accessible fitness options among older adults and individuals with limited mobility. Traditional yoga has long been celebrated for its health benefits, but its physical demands often made it inaccessible to seniors and those with physical limitations. Recognizing this gap, yoga practitioners and therapists began adapting yoga poses to be performed from a seated position, leading to the development of Chair Yoga.

Chair Yoga gained significant attention in the late 20th and early 21st centuries as the population of older adults increased globally. With advancements in healthcare and longer life expectancies, there was a heightened focus on promoting active aging and maintaining physical and mental health among seniors. Chair Yoga became a popular solution, offering a safe and effective way for seniors to stay active without the risks associated with more strenuous forms of exercise.

Over the years, Chair Yoga has evolved to incorporate a wide range of techniques and practices. Early adaptations focused primarily on modifying traditional poses, but contemporary Chair Yoga often integrates elements of meditation, breathing exercises, and relaxation techniques. This holistic approach ensures that practitioners not only improve their physical health but also enhance their mental and emotional well-being.

The evolution of Chair Yoga has also been influenced by research and clinical practice. Studies have demonstrated the numerous benefits of Chair Yoga for seniors, including improved flexibility, reduced pain, enhanced mood, and better overall quality of life. These findings have further validated Chair Yoga as a valuable practice for older adults, leading to its widespread adoption in various settings such as nursing homes, rehabilitation centers, and community classes.

Today, Chair Yoga continues to grow and adapt to the needs of its practitioners. Innovations in teaching methods, the incorporation of technology, and the development of specialized Chair Yoga programs have made it more accessible and effective than ever before. As a result, Chair Yoga has established itself as a vital tool for promoting health and wellness among seniors, helping them lead more active, balanced, and fulfilling lives.

Differences Between Chair Yoga and Traditional Yoga

While Chair Yoga shares many foundational elements with traditional yoga, there are several key differences that make it uniquely suited for seniors and individuals with limited mobility. The most obvious distinction is the use of a chair as a prop, which provides support and stability throughout the practice. This modification allows practitioners to perform yoga poses without the need to stand or kneel, reducing the risk of falls and injuries.

Another significant difference lies in the intensity and complexity of the poses. Traditional yoga often involves a wide range of poses that require varying degrees of strength, flexibility, and balance. In contrast, Chair Yoga focuses on gentle movements and simplified versions of these poses, making them more accessible and manageable for older adults. This adaptation ensures that Chair Yoga remains safe and comfortable for its target audience without compromising the benefits of the practice.

Breathing techniques and meditation are integral to both Chair Yoga and traditional yoga, but their application may differ slightly. In Chair Yoga, breathing exercises are often emphasized to help practitioners relax and connect with their bodies while seated. Meditation practices may also be tailored to accommodate the seated position, allowing for deeper mental relaxation and stress reduction without the physical strain of traditional poses
.

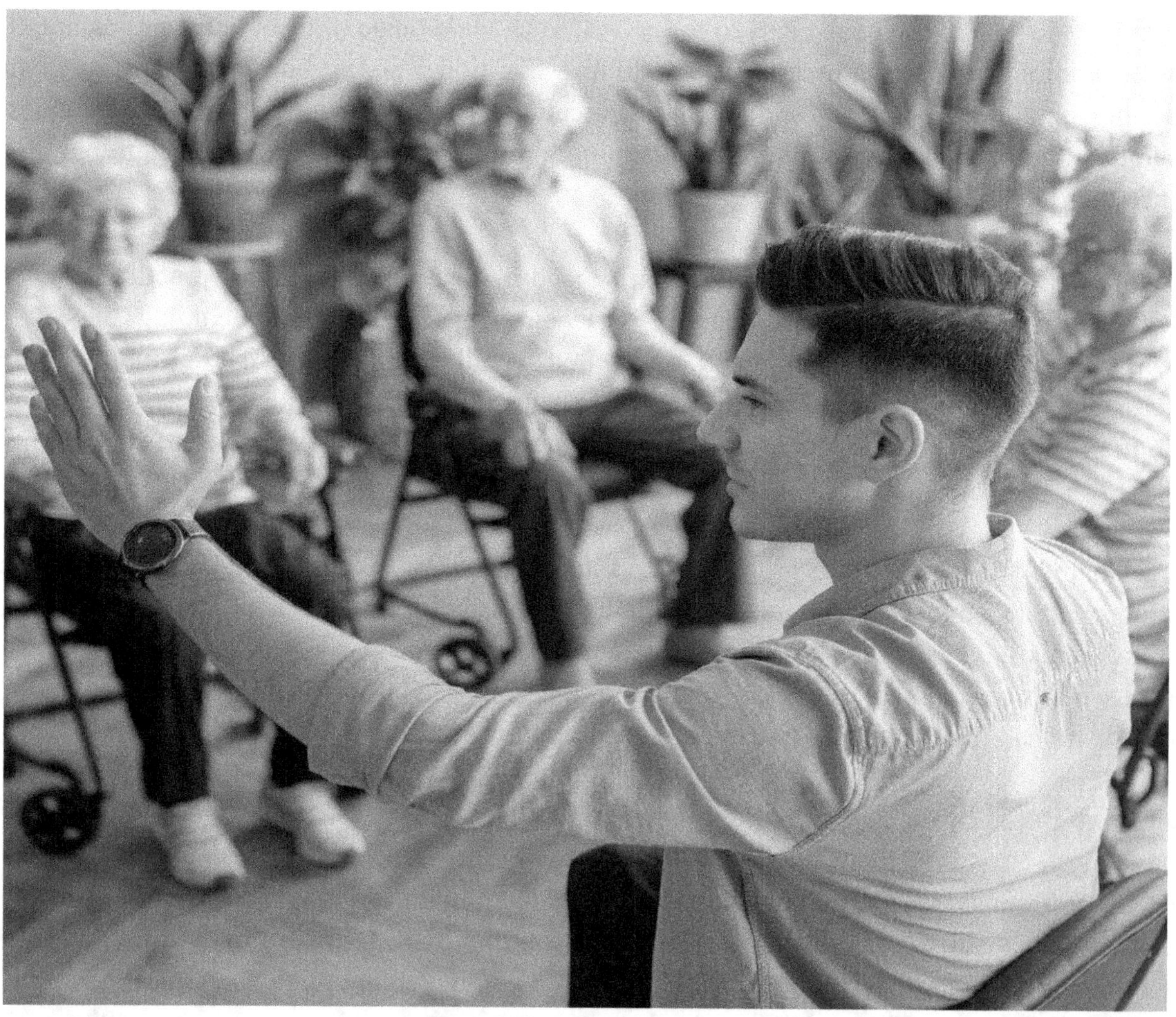

The pace and flow of Chair Yoga sessions also distinguish it from traditional yoga. Chair Yoga typically moves at a slower, more deliberate pace, allowing practitioners to focus on each movement and breath. This slower tempo helps seniors maintain control over their bodies, prevents overexertion, and fosters a sense of mindfulness and presence. Traditional yoga, on the other hand, may involve more dynamic and faster-paced sequences that require greater physical exertion and coordination.

The accessibility and adaptability of Chair Yoga set it apart from traditional yoga. Chair Yoga can be easily modified to accommodate various physical conditions and limitations, making it a versatile practice for a diverse range of individuals. Traditional yoga may require additional props or advanced techniques to achieve similar levels of accessibility, whereas Chair Yoga is inherently designed to be inclusive and adaptable from the outset.

Benefits of Chair Yoga for Seniors

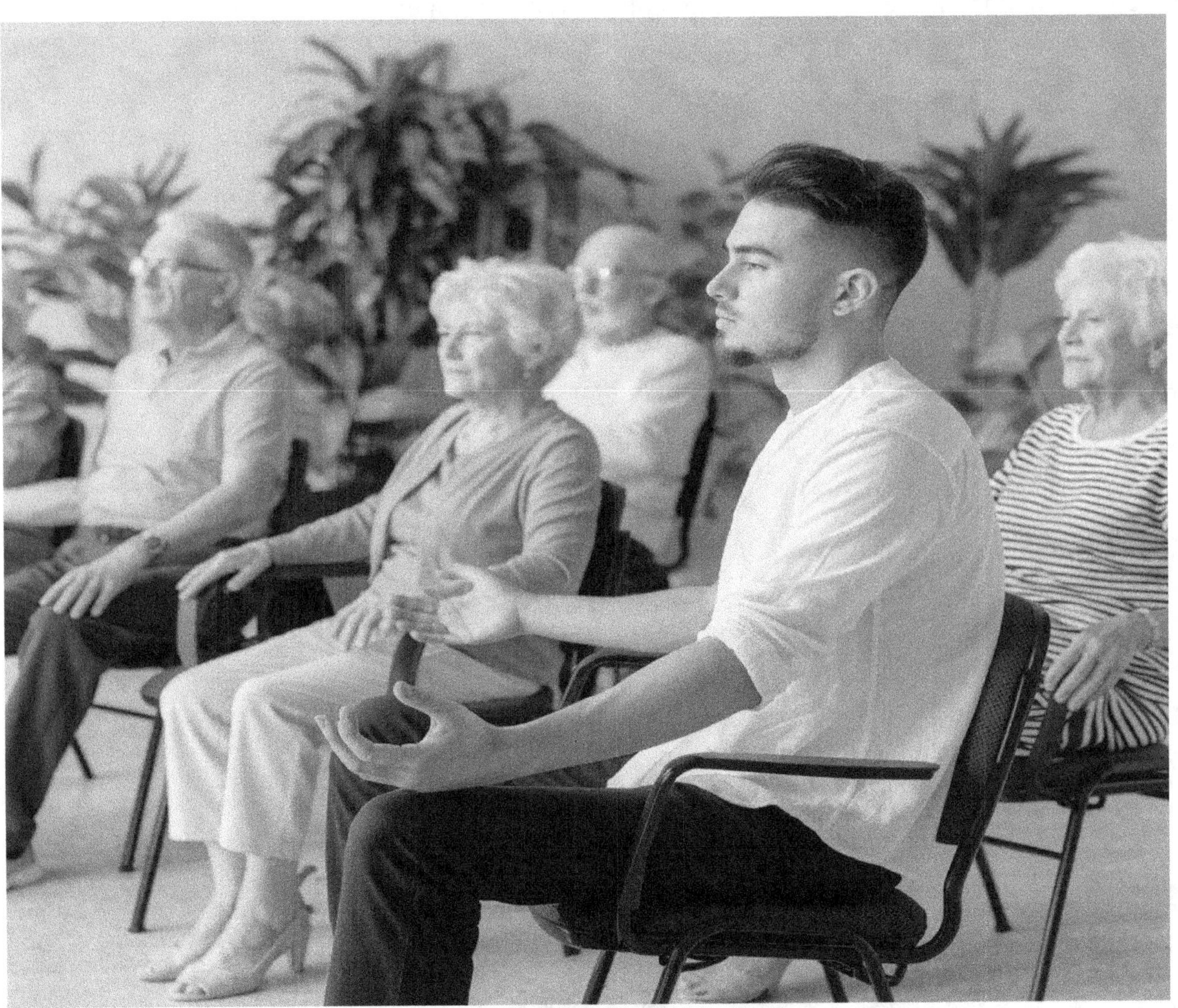

Physical Health Benefits

Chair Yoga offers a multitude of physical health benefits that are particularly valuable for seniors over 70. One of the primary advantages is improved flexibility. As we age, our muscles and joints naturally become stiffer, leading to decreased mobility and increased risk of injury. Chair Yoga incorporates gentle stretching and movement that help maintain and enhance flexibility, making everyday tasks easier and reducing the likelihood of falls.

In addition to flexibility, Chair Yoga contributes to increased strength. Many of the exercises target key muscle groups, including the arms, legs, and core, helping to maintain muscle mass and prevent the muscle loss that commonly occurs with aging. Strengthened muscles provide better support for the joints, reduce pain, and enhance overall stability, which is crucial for maintaining independence and performing daily activities with ease.

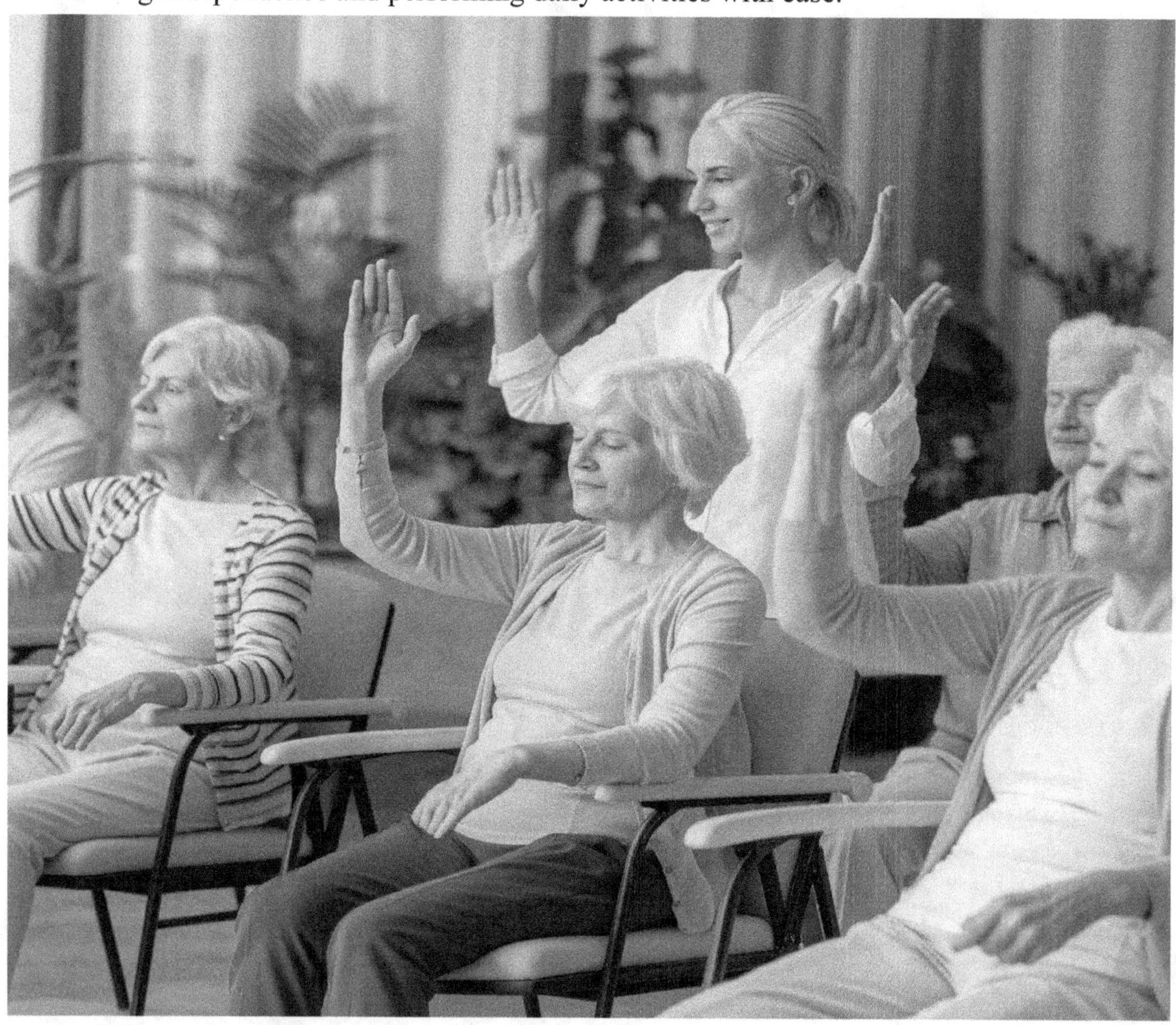

Another significant physical benefit of Chair Yoga is improved circulation. The slow, controlled movements combined with deep breathing exercises help stimulate blood flow throughout the body. Enhanced circulation can lead to better oxygen and nutrient delivery to the tissues, promoting healing and overall health. Improved circulation also aids in the prevention of conditions such as hypertension and cardiovascular disease, which are prevalent among older adults.

Chair Yoga also supports joint health by reducing stiffness and increasing the range of motion. Regular practice can alleviate symptoms of arthritis and other joint-related issues, allowing seniors to move more comfortably and with less pain. By keeping the joints mobile and lubricated, Chair Yoga helps prevent the degeneration of cartilage and reduces the impact of chronic conditions on daily life.

Chair Yoga can contribute to weight management. While it may not be as intense as other forms of exercise, the combination of movement and mindfulness can help regulate appetite and improve metabolic function. Engaging in Chair Yoga regularly encourages a more active lifestyle, which, when combined with proper nutrition, can help seniors maintain a healthy weight and reduce the risk of obesity-related diseases.

Mental and Emotional Well-being

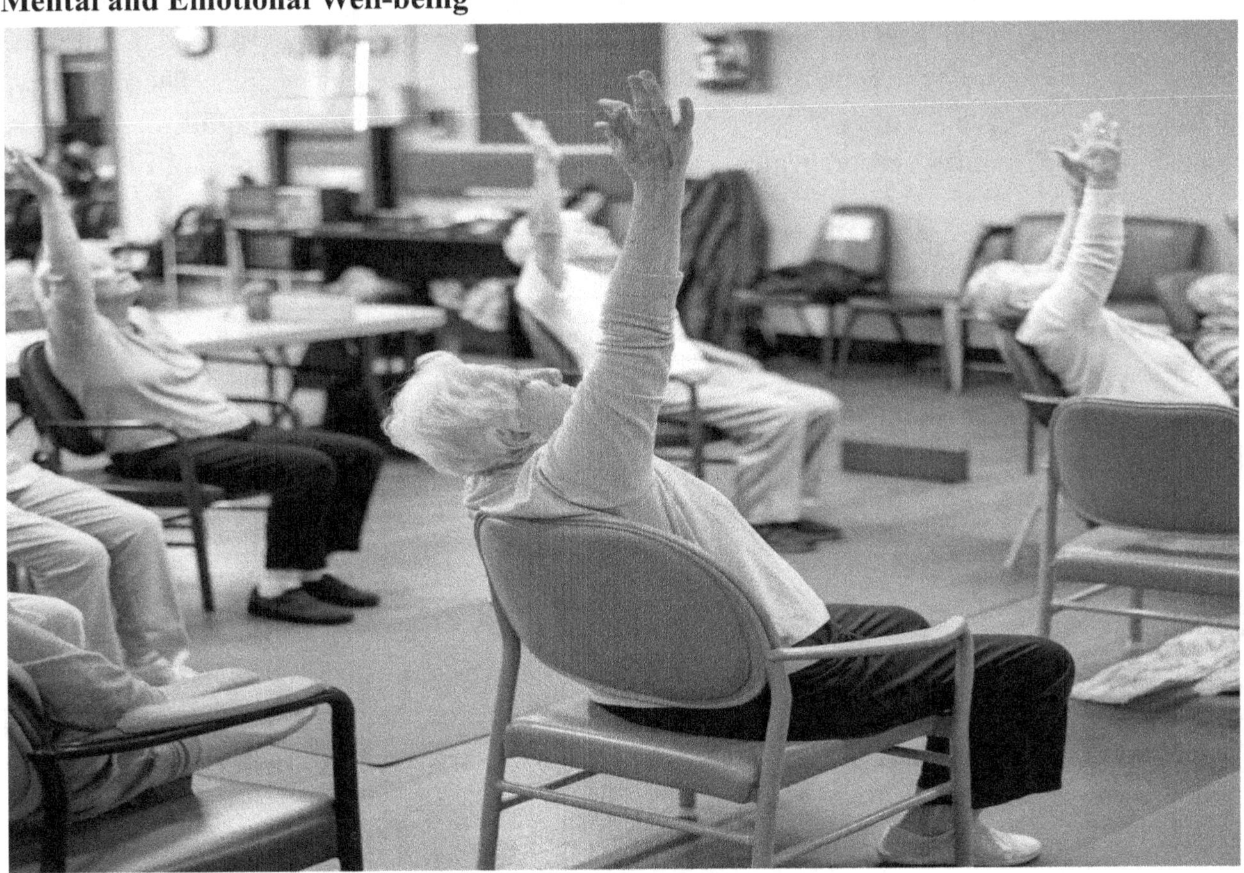

Beyond the physical advantages, Chair Yoga offers profound mental and emotional benefits that enhance the overall quality of life for seniors. One of the most notable benefits is stress reduction. The combination of deep breathing, meditation, and mindful movement helps activate the body's relaxation response, lowering cortisol levels and promoting a sense of calm and tranquility. This is especially beneficial for seniors who may experience anxiety or stress related to health concerns or life changes.

Chair Yoga also enhances mental clarity and cognitive function. Engaging in regular practice stimulates the brain, improving memory, concentration, and overall mental sharpness. The focus required during yoga sessions helps keep the mind active and engaged, which can be particularly beneficial in preventing cognitive decline and diseases such as Alzheimer's.

Emotional well-being is another key area where Chair Yoga makes a significant impact. The practice fosters a sense of accomplishment and self-efficacy, as seniors successfully perform poses and complete routines tailored to their abilities. This boost in confidence can lead to improved self-esteem and a more positive outlook on life. Additionally, the meditative aspects of Chair Yoga encourage introspection and emotional balance, helping individuals manage feelings of sadness or loneliness.

Social interaction is also facilitated through Chair Yoga, whether practiced in group settings or classes. Engaging with peers who share similar interests fosters a sense of community and belonging, combating feelings of isolation that are common among older adults. The supportive environment of Chair Yoga classes provides opportunities for meaningful connections, friendships, and mutual encouragement, all of which contribute to emotional resilience and happiness.

Furthermore, Chair Yoga promotes better sleep patterns. The relaxation techniques and physical activity involved in the practice help regulate sleep cycles, making it easier for seniors to fall asleep and enjoy restful, uninterrupted sleep. Improved sleep quality enhances overall health, mood, and cognitive function, allowing seniors to wake up feeling refreshed and energized each day.

Social and Community Advantages

Chair Yoga not only benefits individuals on a personal level but also fosters a sense of community and social connection among seniors. Participating in Chair Yoga classes or groups provides an opportunity for social interaction, which is essential for emotional health and combating loneliness. Engaging with others in a shared activity helps build friendships and a support network, enhancing the overall quality of life.

In group settings, Chair Yoga encourages teamwork and mutual support. Seniors can motivate each other, share experiences, and celebrate progress together. This collective effort creates a positive and uplifting environment where individuals feel valued and connected. The social aspect of Chair Yoga classes can lead to lasting relationships and a stronger sense of community belonging.

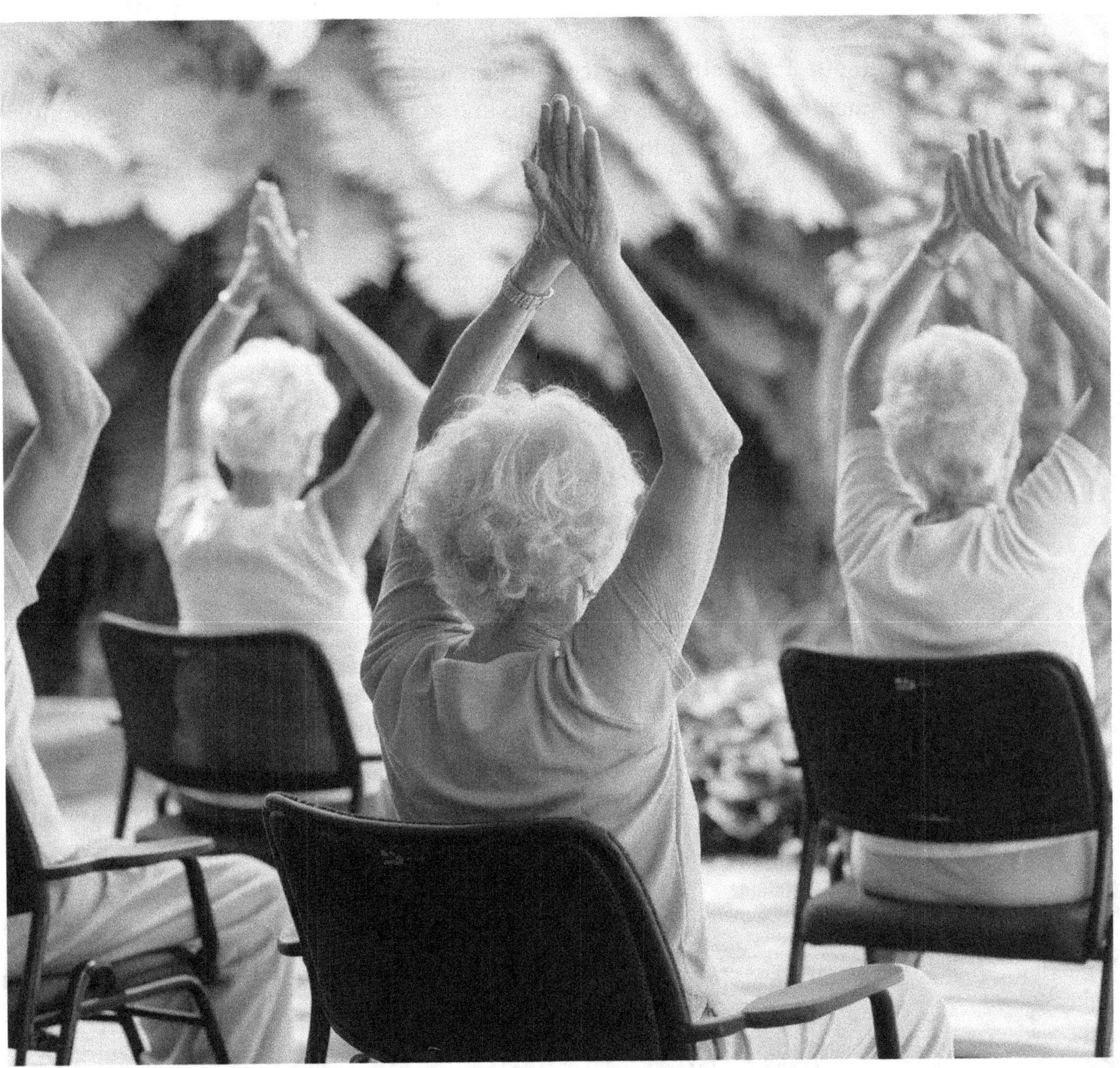

Moreover, Chair Yoga can serve as a gateway to broader community involvement. As seniors become more active and confident through their practice, they may be inspired to participate in other social or recreational activities. This increased engagement can lead to greater community involvement, volunteering opportunities, and participation in local events, further enriching their lives and fostering a sense of purpose.

Chair Yoga also provides a platform for intergenerational interaction. Families and caregivers can join seniors in their practice, promoting bonding and understanding across generations. This shared activity strengthens family ties and creates meaningful moments of connection and support, enhancing the emotional well-being of both seniors and their loved ones.

Chair Yoga contributes to the creation of inclusive and supportive communities. By offering a practice that accommodates varying physical abilities, Chair Yoga promotes diversity and accessibility within fitness and wellness spaces. This inclusivity ensures that all individuals, regardless of their physical condition, can participate and benefit from yoga, fostering a culture of acceptance and mutual respect within the community.

How to Use This Book

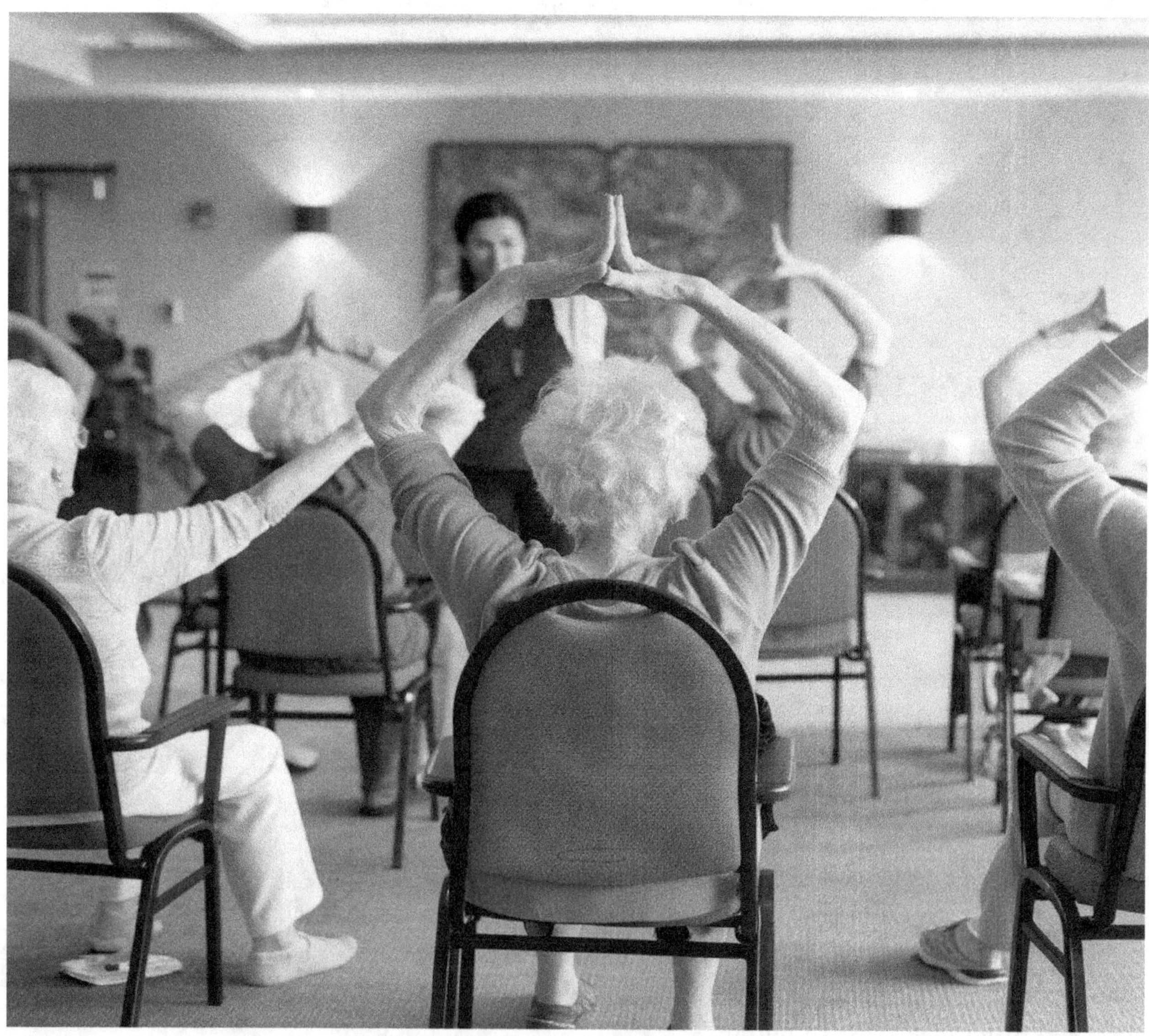

Navigating the Chapters

This book is structured to provide a comprehensive guide to Chair Yoga for seniors over 70, with each chapter building upon the previous one to create a cohesive and effective practice. To navigate the chapters effectively, it is recommended to start with the introductory chapters that lay the foundation of Chair Yoga, including its definitions, benefits, and how to prepare for your practice. These sections offer essential knowledge that will enhance your understanding and maximize the benefits you receive from the exercises.

Each subsequent chapter delves into specific aspects of Chair Yoga, such as breathing techniques, strength training, flexibility, and meditation. The chapters are organized logically, allowing you to progress at your own pace. Whether you prefer to follow the book sequentially or focus on particular areas of interest, the clear structure ensures that you can easily find the information and exercises that best meet your needs.

Additionally, this book includes practical tips and guidelines throughout each chapter to help you integrate Chair Yoga into your daily routine. From setting up your practice space to selecting the right chair, these tips provide actionable steps that make it easier to incorporate yoga into your life. By following the organized flow of the book, you can create a personalized Chair Yoga practice that aligns with your health goals and lifestyle.

To further enhance your experience, this book features illustrations and descriptions of each pose, making it simple to follow along even if you are new to yoga. Detailed instructions and modifications are provided to ensure that each exercise is performed safely and effectively. This visual and descriptive approach allows you to practice confidently, knowing that you have clear guidance every step of the way.

Moreover, this book includes summaries and key takeaways at the end of each chapter, reinforcing the main points and helping you retain the information. These summaries serve as quick references that you can revisit whenever needed, ensuring that you have a solid grasp of the concepts and techniques discussed. By utilizing the structured layout and comprehensive content, you can fully engage with the book and achieve the best possible results from your Chair Yoga practice.

Tips for Maximizing Benefits

To fully experience the benefits of Chair Yoga, it is important to approach your practice with intention and consistency. One of the key tips for maximizing benefits is to establish a regular practice schedule. Consistency helps to reinforce the habits and movements, allowing your body and mind to adapt and respond positively over time. Setting aside dedicated time each day or several times a week ensures that Chair Yoga becomes an integral part of your routine.

Another important tip is to listen to your body and respect your limits. While Chair Yoga is designed to be gentle, it is essential to pay attention to how your body feels during each exercise. Avoid pushing yourself beyond your comfort level, and make modifications as needed to ensure that each movement is performed safely. By tuning into your body's signals, you can prevent injuries and make your practice more enjoyable and effective.

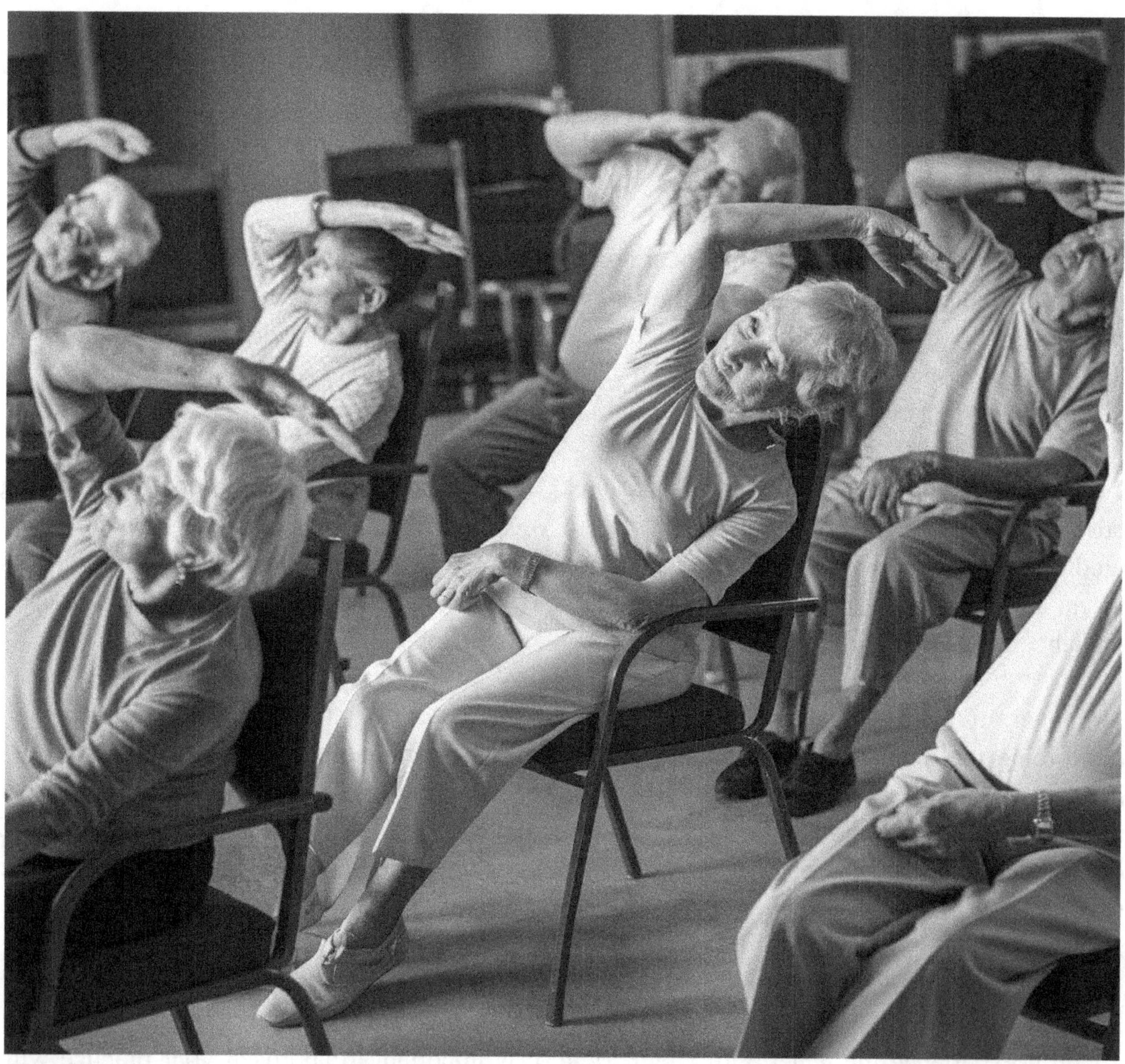

Creating a conducive environment for your practice is also crucial. Choose a quiet, comfortable space where you can focus without distractions. Ensure that your chair is stable and provides adequate support, and consider adding cushions or props to enhance comfort. A well-prepared space can significantly enhance your practice, making it easier to relax and concentrate on your movements and breathing.

Incorporating mindful breathing and relaxation techniques can further enhance the benefits of Chair Yoga. Focused breathing helps to calm the mind, reduce stress, and improve oxygen flow throughout the body. Taking the time to breathe deeply and mindfully during each session can amplify the physical benefits and contribute to a greater sense of mental clarity and emotional balance.

Setting personal goals can provide motivation and direction for your practice. Whether you aim to increase flexibility, reduce pain, or enhance mental well-being, having clear objectives helps you stay focused and track your progress. Reflecting on your goals regularly and adjusting them as needed ensures that your Chair Yoga practice remains aligned with your evolving needs and aspirations, leading to sustained benefits and a more fulfilling experience.

Setting Personal Goals

Setting personal goals is a fundamental aspect of your Chair Yoga journey, providing direction and purpose to your practice. Begin by identifying what you hope to achieve through Chair Yoga, whether it's improving physical health, enhancing flexibility, reducing stress, or fostering social connections. Clear goals help you stay motivated and focused, ensuring that your practice remains meaningful and aligned with your personal needs and aspirations.

When setting goals, it is important to make them specific, measurable, achievable, relevant, and time-bound (SMART). For example, instead of setting a vague goal like "improve flexibility," aim for something more concrete, such as "increase the range of motion in my shoulders within three months." This approach allows you to track your progress effectively and stay committed to your objectives, making it easier to celebrate milestones along the way.

In addition to physical goals, consider incorporating mental and emotional objectives into your Chair Yoga practice. Goals such as reducing anxiety, enhancing mindfulness, or improving sleep quality can significantly contribute to your overall well-being. By addressing both physical and mental aspects, you create a holistic approach to health that maximizes the benefits of Chair Yoga and supports a balanced, fulfilling life.It is also beneficial to periodically review and adjust your goals as you progress in your practice. As you achieve certain milestones, you may find that your needs and aspirations evolve. Regularly reassessing your goals ensures that your Chair Yoga practice remains dynamic and responsive to your changing circumstances, allowing you to continue growing and experiencing new benefits over time.

Sharing your goals with a trusted friend, family member, or yoga instructor can provide additional support and accountability. Having someone to encourage you and celebrate your achievements can enhance your motivation and commitment to your practice. By setting thoughtful, personalized goals and actively working towards them, you can fully embrace the transformative potential of Chair Yoga and enjoy a healthier, happier life.

Chapter 2

GETTING STARTED

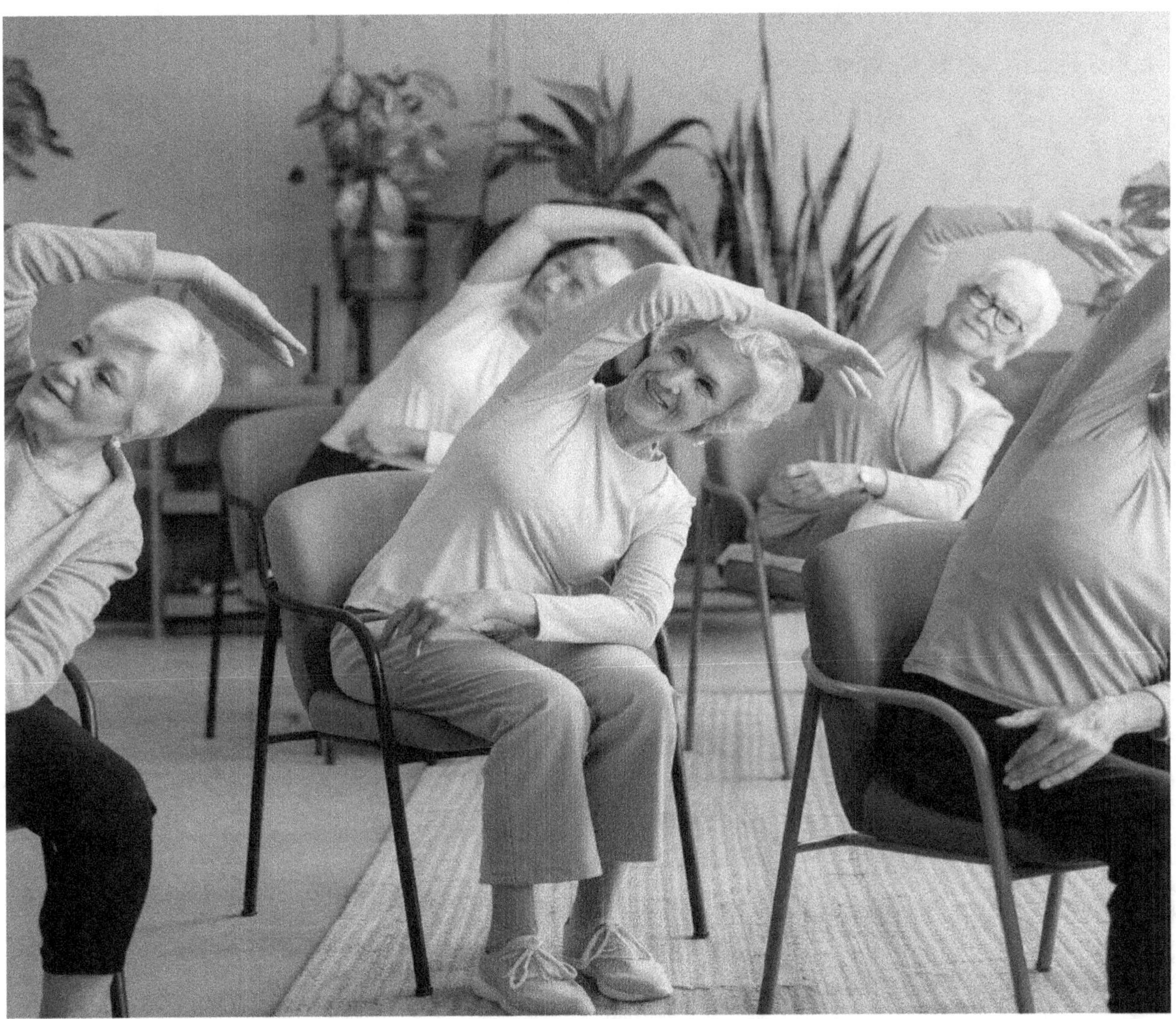

Embarking on your 30-day stretching journey is an exciting first step toward enhanced health and vitality, especially tailored for seniors seeking to improve their flexibility, strength, and overall well-being. In this chapter, I lay the foundation for your success by guiding you through essential preparations, from creating a comfortable and safe exercise space to understanding the basic principles of effective stretching. You'll learn how to set realistic goals, track your progress, and listen to your body's signals to prevent injury and ensure a positive experience. Additionally, I'll provide valuable tips on selecting the right attire and any necessary equipment, as well as strategies to stay motivated and consistent throughout the program. Whether you're new to stretching or returning after a hiatus, this chapter equips you with the knowledge and confidence to begin your transformative journey with ease and assurance. Let's take the first step together towards a healthier, more flexible, and stronger you.

Preparing Your Space

Choosing the Right Environment

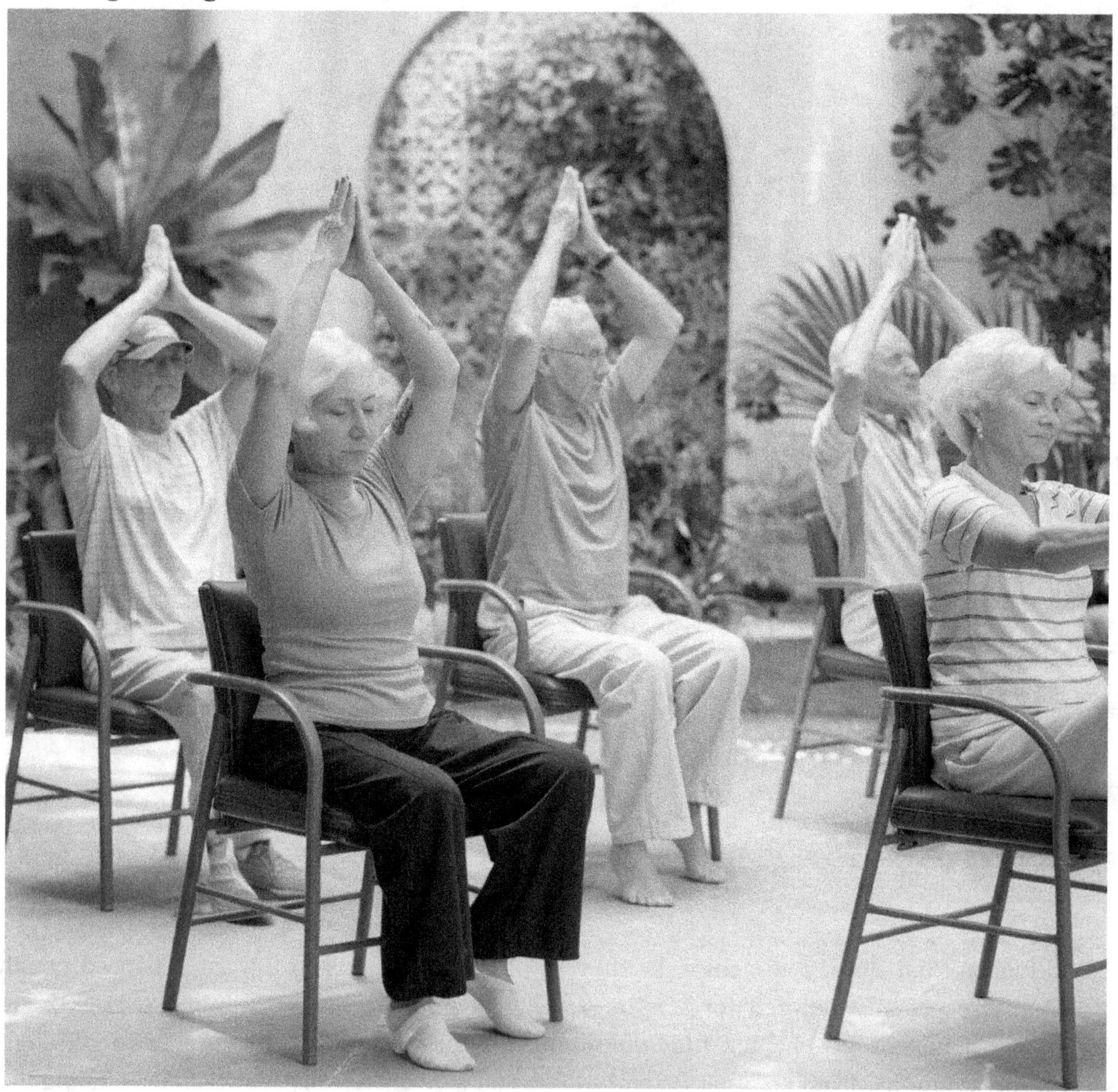

Creating an ideal environment is the first step toward a successful chair yoga practice. Select a quiet and peaceful area in your home where you can focus without distractions. Natural light and good ventilation can enhance your mood and energy levels, making your yoga session more enjoyable. Ensure that the space is free from clutter, as a tidy area promotes a clear mind and reduces the risk of tripping or stumbling during exercises.

Consider the temperature of the room as well. A comfortable, moderately warm environment helps your muscles relax and prevents stiffness. If the space tends to be cold, you might use a portable heater or have a blanket nearby to stay warm. Conversely, if the room is too warm, ensure adequate ventilation to maintain a comfortable temperature throughout your practice.

Lighting plays a significant role in setting the right atmosphere. Soft, natural lighting is preferable, as it creates a calm and inviting space. If natural light is limited, use lamps with warm bulbs to mimic daylight without being harsh on the eyes. Proper lighting not only enhances your mood but also allows you to see your movements clearly, reducing the chances of misalignment.

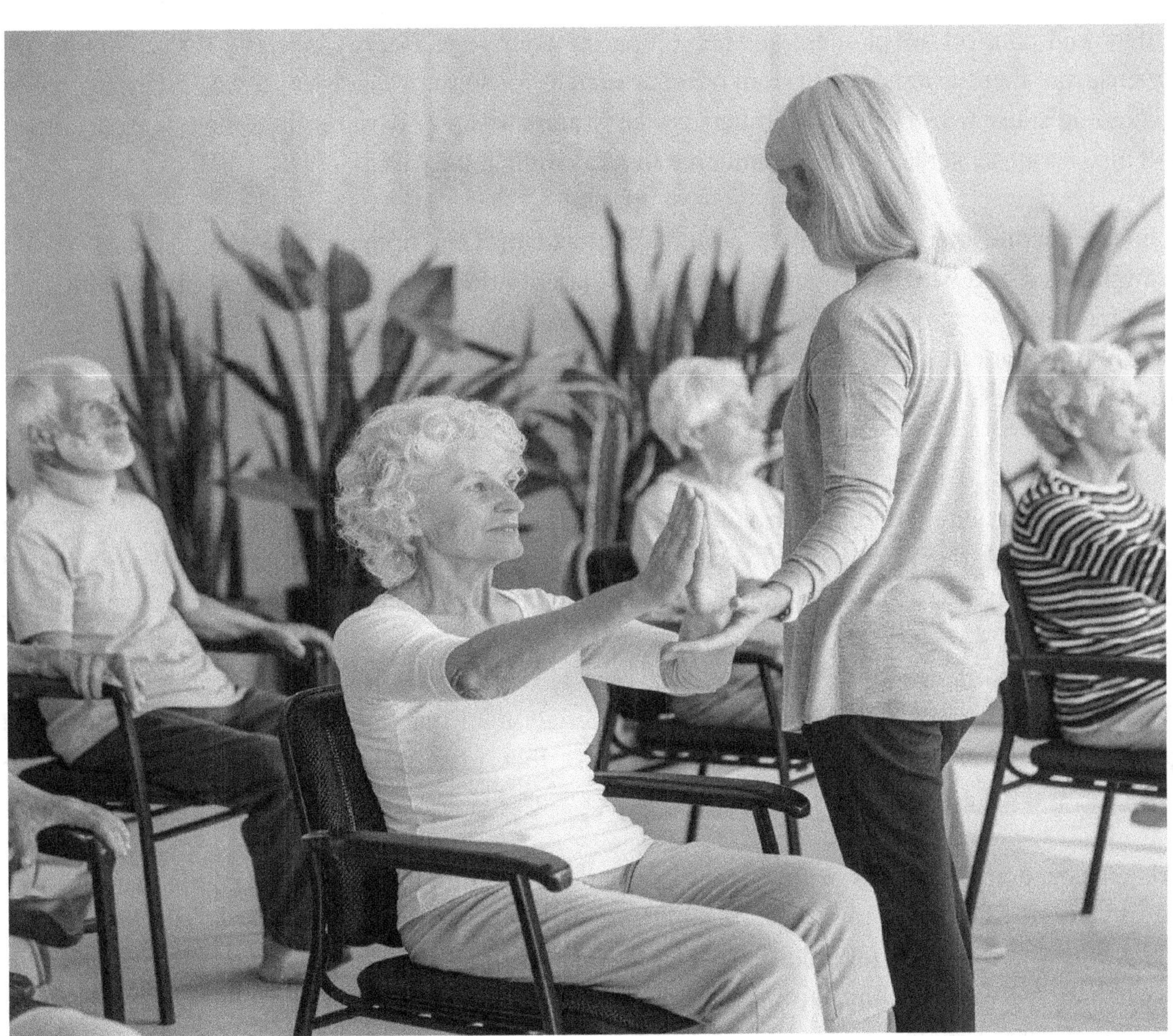

Incorporate elements that promote relaxation and focus, such as soothing music, scented candles, or essential oil diffusers. Gentle background music can help you stay centered and maintain a steady rhythm during your practice. However, ensure that the volume is low enough not to be distracting. Aromatherapy with calming scents like lavender or eucalyptus can further enhance your sense of well-being.

Personalize your yoga space to make it inviting and motivating. Adding personal touches like plants, artwork, or inspirational quotes can create a positive environment that encourages regular practice. A dedicated yoga area serves as a visual reminder of your commitment to health and wellness, making it easier to integrate chair yoga into your daily routine.

Ensuring Safety and Comfort

Safety and comfort are paramount when preparing your yoga space, especially for seniors. Begin by ensuring that the area is free from hazards such as loose rugs, electrical cords, or sharp objects that could cause trips or falls. A clutter-free environment not only minimizes the risk of accidents but also creates a serene setting conducive to relaxation and focus.

Choose a comfortable chair with a sturdy base to prevent tipping. The chair should have a straight back and be free of wheels to provide stability during exercises. Avoid chairs with arms that are too low or too high, as they can interfere with your movements. If your chair has arms, ensure they are wide enough to allow free movement of your arms during stretching and strengthening exercises.

Consider using a non-slip mat or placing the chair on a stable surface to enhance grip and prevent sliding. Non-slip mats provide additional traction, especially if your legs are slick from movement or if the floor is hardwood or tile. Ensuring that your feet remain firmly planted during exercises is crucial for maintaining balance and executing movements safely.

Dress in comfortable, loose-fitting clothing that allows for a full range of motion. Breathable fabrics such as cotton or moisture-wicking materials help regulate your body temperature and prevent overheating. Avoid restrictive garments that may limit your movements or cause discomfort during stretching and strengthening exercises.

Also, keep essential items within reach to maintain comfort and safety. Have a water bottle nearby to stay hydrated, and keep a small towel handy to wipe away sweat if necessary. A blanket can be useful for additional warmth or support during relaxation periods. Having everything you need within arm's reach ensures that you can focus entirely on your practice without unnecessary interruptions.

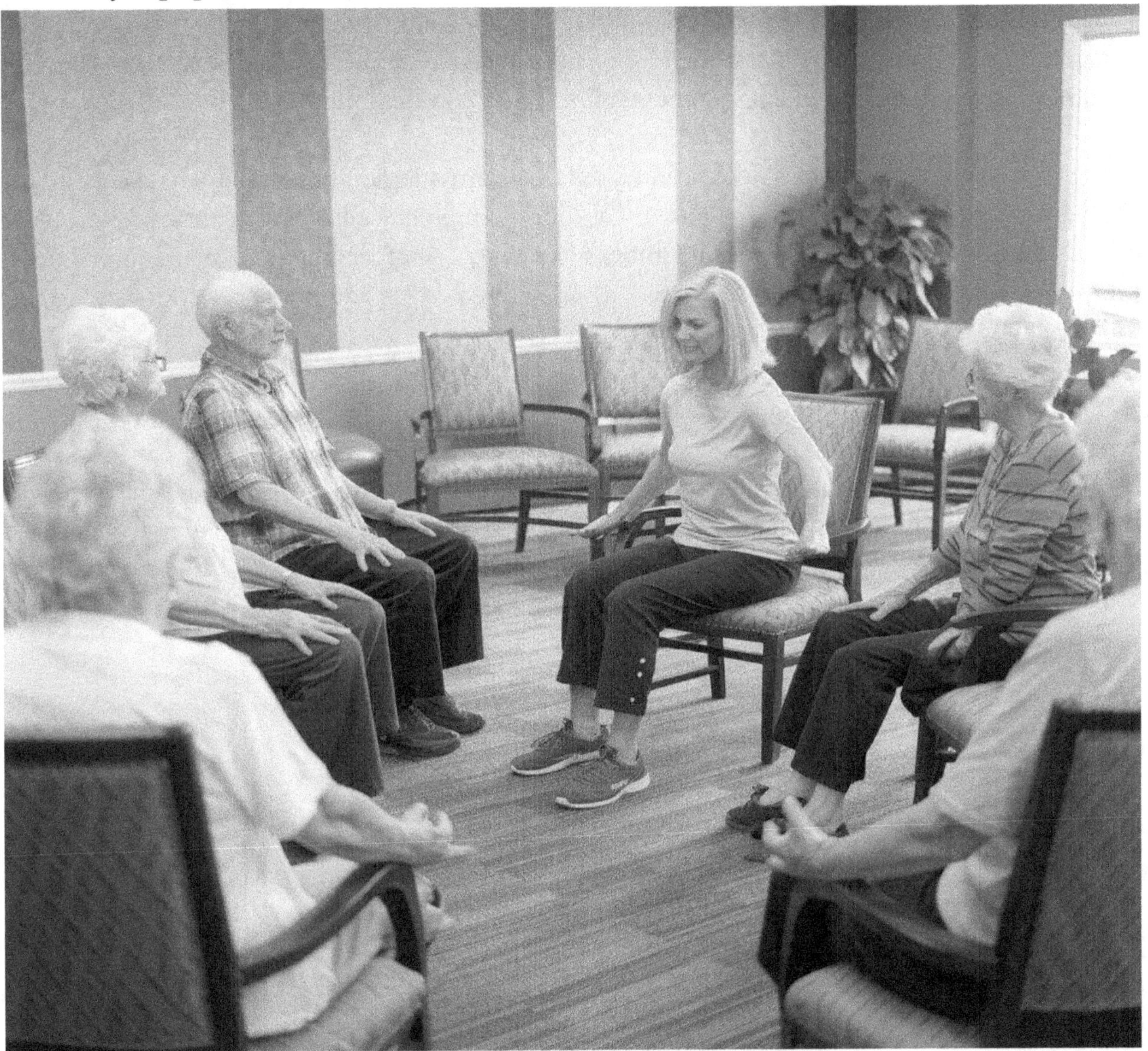

While chair yoga requires minimal equipment, having the right accessories can enhance your practice and provide additional support. A sturdy, comfortable chair is the most essential piece of equipment. As previously mentioned, ensure that the chair is stable, has a straight back, and is free of wheels. This will provide the necessary support for various poses and movements.

A yoga mat is beneficial for providing cushioning and support, especially if your chair does not have adequate padding. Place the mat on the floor beneath your chair to prevent slipping and to add a layer of comfort for your feet and legs. Mats also help define your practice space, creating a mental boundary that signals the start of your yoga session.

Resistance bands are a versatile tool that can be incorporated into your chair yoga routine to add strength training elements. They are lightweight, portable, and come in various resistance levels to match your strength and fitness goals. Resistance bands can be used for exercises targeting different muscle groups, enhancing your overall strength and flexibility.

Yoga props such as cushions, blocks, and straps can provide additional support and help you achieve proper alignment in various poses. Cushions can be placed behind your back for added support during seated stretches, while blocks can assist in reaching and maintaining poses comfortably. Straps help extend your reach, allowing you to engage in deeper stretches without straining.

I want you to know that having a timer or a clock nearby can help you manage the duration of your sessions and ensure that you are pacing yourself appropriately. A timer can be set for specific exercises or relaxation periods, keeping your practice organized and efficient. Additionally, keeping a journal to note your progress, feelings, and any challenges can be a valuable tool for tracking your journey and staying motivated.

Selecting the Right Chair

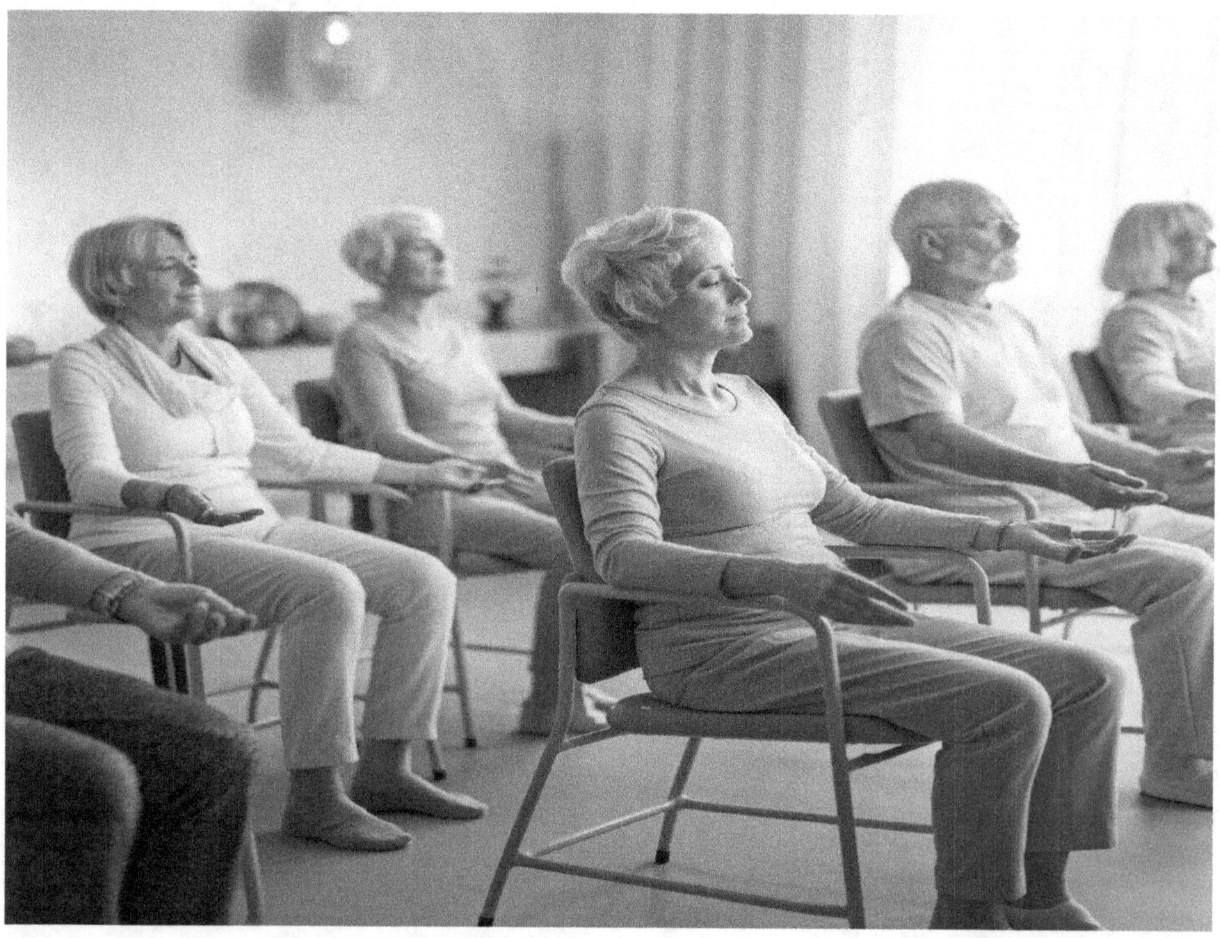

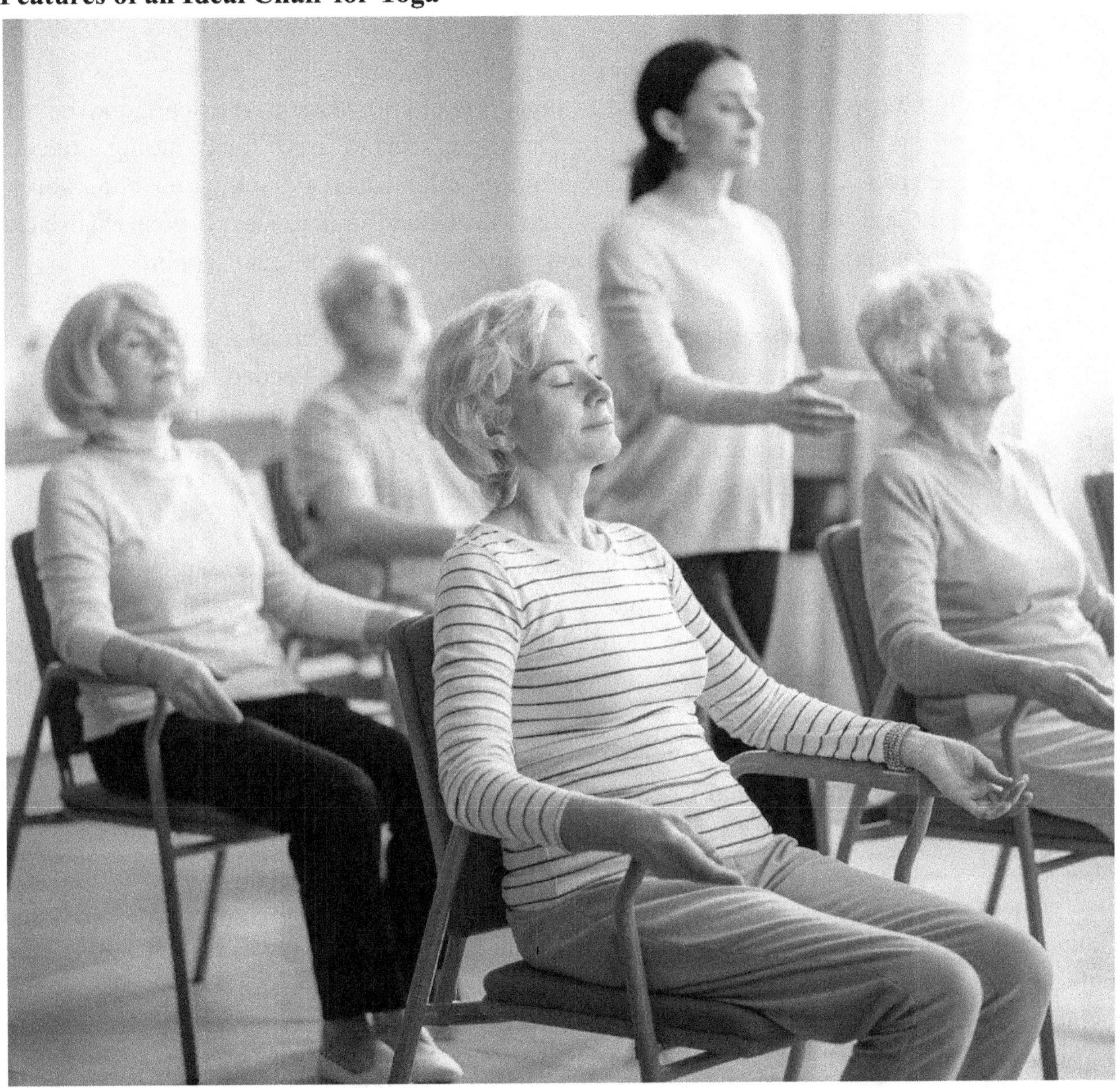

Selecting the right chair is crucial for a safe and effective chair yoga practice. An ideal yoga chair should be sturdy and stable, with a solid base to prevent tipping or wobbling during movements. Chairs with a broad, flat base provide better support and balance, allowing you to perform various exercises with confidence. Avoid chairs with wheels or those that are easily movable, as they can compromise stability and increase the risk of falls.

Comfort is another essential feature of a suitable yoga chair. The chair should have a straight, supportive back that encourages proper posture and alignment. A cushioned seat can enhance comfort, especially during longer sessions, but it should not be too soft, as this can make it difficult to maintain proper support. Ensure that the chair's height is adjustable or matches your natural seated height, allowing your feet to rest flat on the floor with your knees at a 90-degree angle.

Armrests should be appropriately positioned to support your arms without restricting movement. Ideally, the armrests should be wide enough to allow your arms to move freely during stretches and strength exercises. Chairs with adjustable armrests offer added flexibility, enabling you to modify the height and width to suit your individual needs and preferences. If your chair lacks armrests, consider adding detachable ones or using yoga straps for additional support.

The material of the chair also plays a role in your comfort and mobility. Chairs made of lightweight materials such as wood or plastic are easier to move if needed, while upholstered chairs provide additional cushioning for comfort. However, ensure that the upholstery is durable and easy to clean, as regular use can lead to wear and tear. Breathable fabrics can help regulate your body temperature, preventing discomfort during your practice.

Consider the overall design and aesthetics of the chair. A chair that resonates with your personal style and preferences can make your yoga space more inviting and enjoyable. Whether you prefer a modern, minimalist design or a more traditional, ornate style, choosing a chair that you find visually appealing can enhance your motivation and commitment to your chair yoga practice.

Adjusting Your Chair for Optimal Use

Once you have selected the right chair, adjusting it properly is essential to maximize comfort and effectiveness during your yoga sessions. Begin by ensuring that the chair is at the correct height relative to your body. Your feet should rest flat on the floor with your knees bent at a 90-degree angle. If the chair is too high, use a footstool or a sturdy cushion to achieve the proper positioning. Conversely, if the chair is too low, consider using thicker cushions or a chair riser to raise it to the appropriate height.

Adjust the backrest to support your spine's natural curve. The back of the chair should align with the small of your back, providing gentle support without forcing you into an unnatural posture. If your chair has an adjustable backrest, modify it to suit your comfort level. For chairs without adjustable backs, you can use a small pillow or cushion to support your lower back, ensuring that your spine remains straight and well-aligned during exercises.

Position the armrests to allow free movement of your arms during stretches and strength training. The armrests should be at a height where your shoulders remain relaxed and do not hunch or elevate during exercises. If your chair's armrests are fixed and do not allow for adjustment, you can use yoga straps or resistance bands to provide additional support and flexibility for your arms, enabling you to perform a wider range of movements comfortably.

Ensure that the chair is placed on a stable, non-slip surface to prevent shifting or sliding during your practice. If your chair tends to move, place a non-slip mat or rug beneath it to enhance stability. This not only provides a secure base but also helps to keep your feet in place, allowing for more effective and controlled movements. Additionally, check that the chair's legs are evenly positioned to maintain balance and prevent tipping.

Finally, make any necessary adjustments to the surrounding environment to support your practice. Arrange any yoga props, such as cushions, blocks, or resistance bands, within easy reach. Ensure that there is enough space around the chair to allow for full arm and leg movements without obstruction. A well-adjusted chair and a thoughtfully arranged space contribute to a comfortable and effective chair yoga session, enhancing your overall experience and results.

Alternatives to Standard Chairs

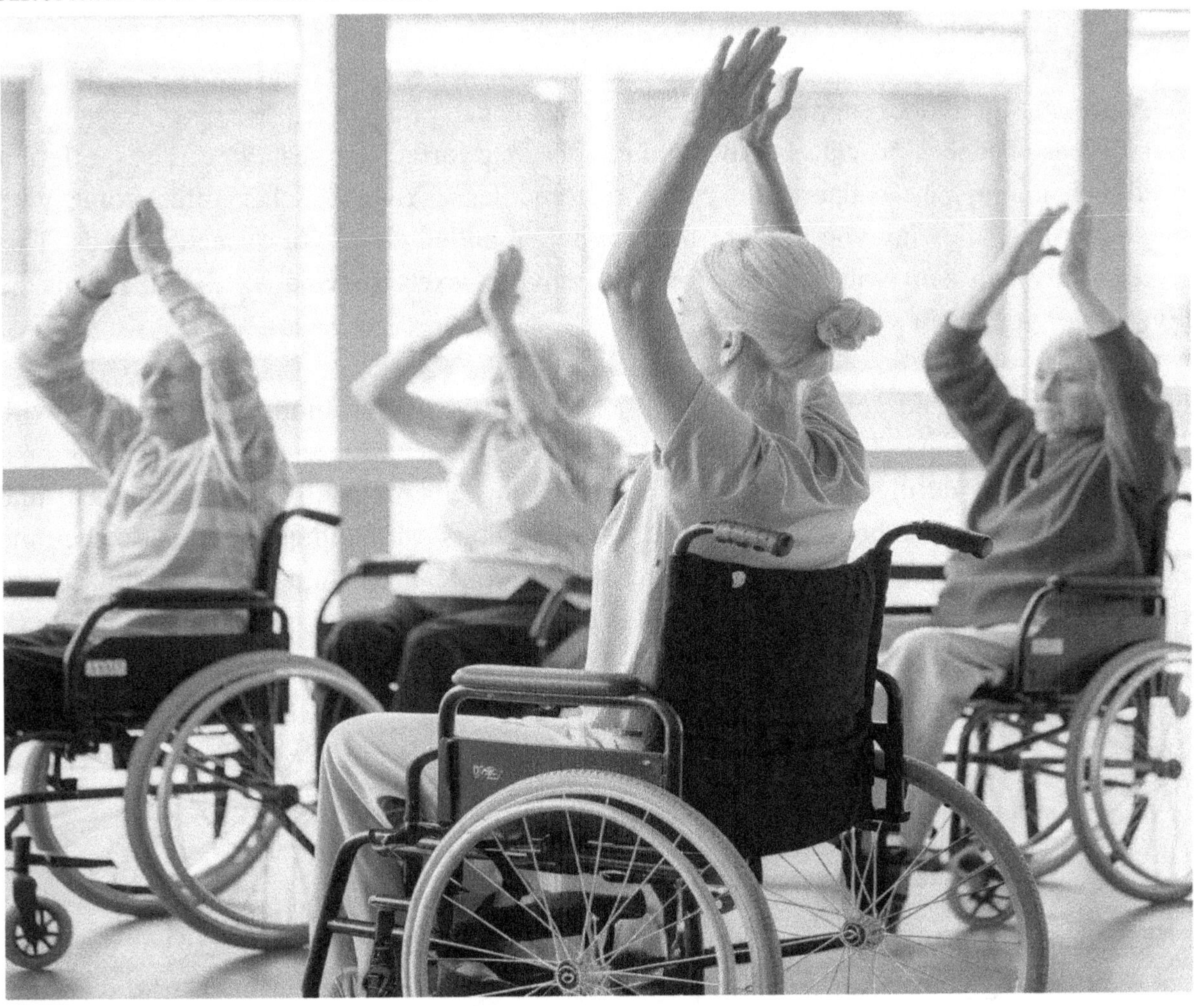

While a standard chair can be perfectly suitable for chair yoga, exploring alternative seating options can provide additional support and versatility to your practice. One popular alternative is the yoga chair, specifically designed for yoga and exercise purposes. Yoga chairs often feature a more ergonomic design with adjustable components to better support various poses and movements. These chairs may include built-in handles or straps, allowing for enhanced grip and assistance during stretching and strength exercises.

Another alternative is the use of a sturdy, high-backed dining chair or an armchair with wide armrests. These chairs provide additional support for your back and arms, making it easier to perform certain yoga poses. High-backed chairs offer better lumbar support, helping to maintain proper spinal alignment during your practice. Additionally, chairs with wide armrests allow for greater flexibility in arm movements, facilitating a wider range of exercises.

Stools can also be used as an alternative to traditional chairs, especially for exercises that require a lower seat height or different angles. Adjustable-height stools provide flexibility, allowing you to modify the seat height to match your comfort and the specific requirements of each exercise. Stools without armrests can offer more freedom of movement for your legs and hips, enabling a greater variety of stretching and strengthening activities.

For those seeking additional support, the use of a yoga bench or a padded exercise bench can be beneficial. These benches provide a stable and comfortable surface for seated exercises, offering enhanced cushioning and support for your back and legs. Yoga benches often come with adjustable features, allowing you to tailor the seat height and angle to your specific needs. This added versatility can help you explore a broader range of exercises and poses, enhancing the effectiveness of your chair yoga practice.

Consider using specialized yoga props such as bolsters or wedge cushions in conjunction with your chair. These props can be placed behind your back or under your legs to provide additional support and comfort during certain poses. Bolsters can help maintain proper alignment and relieve pressure on specific body parts, while wedge cushions can facilitate deeper stretches and enhance flexibility. By incorporating these alternatives, you can create a more customized and supportive chair yoga experience that caters to your individual needs and preferences.

Safety Guidelines

Understanding Your Limits

Prioritizing safety is crucial in any exercise regimen, especially for seniors engaging in chair yoga. Understanding and respecting your physical limits ensures that you perform exercises without overexerting yourself or risking injury. Begin by assessing your current fitness level and any existing health conditions that may affect your ability to perform certain movements. Consulting with a healthcare professional before starting a new exercise program is highly recommended to identify any specific limitations or precautions you should take.

Listen to your body's signals during your yoga practice. Pay attention to how your muscles feel and be mindful of any discomfort or pain that arises. Discomfort is a natural part of stretching and strengthening, but sharp pain is a warning sign that something may be wrong. If you experience pain, ease back from the movement and modify the exercise to a more comfortable position. Pushing through pain can lead to strains or other injuries, hindering your progress and well-being.

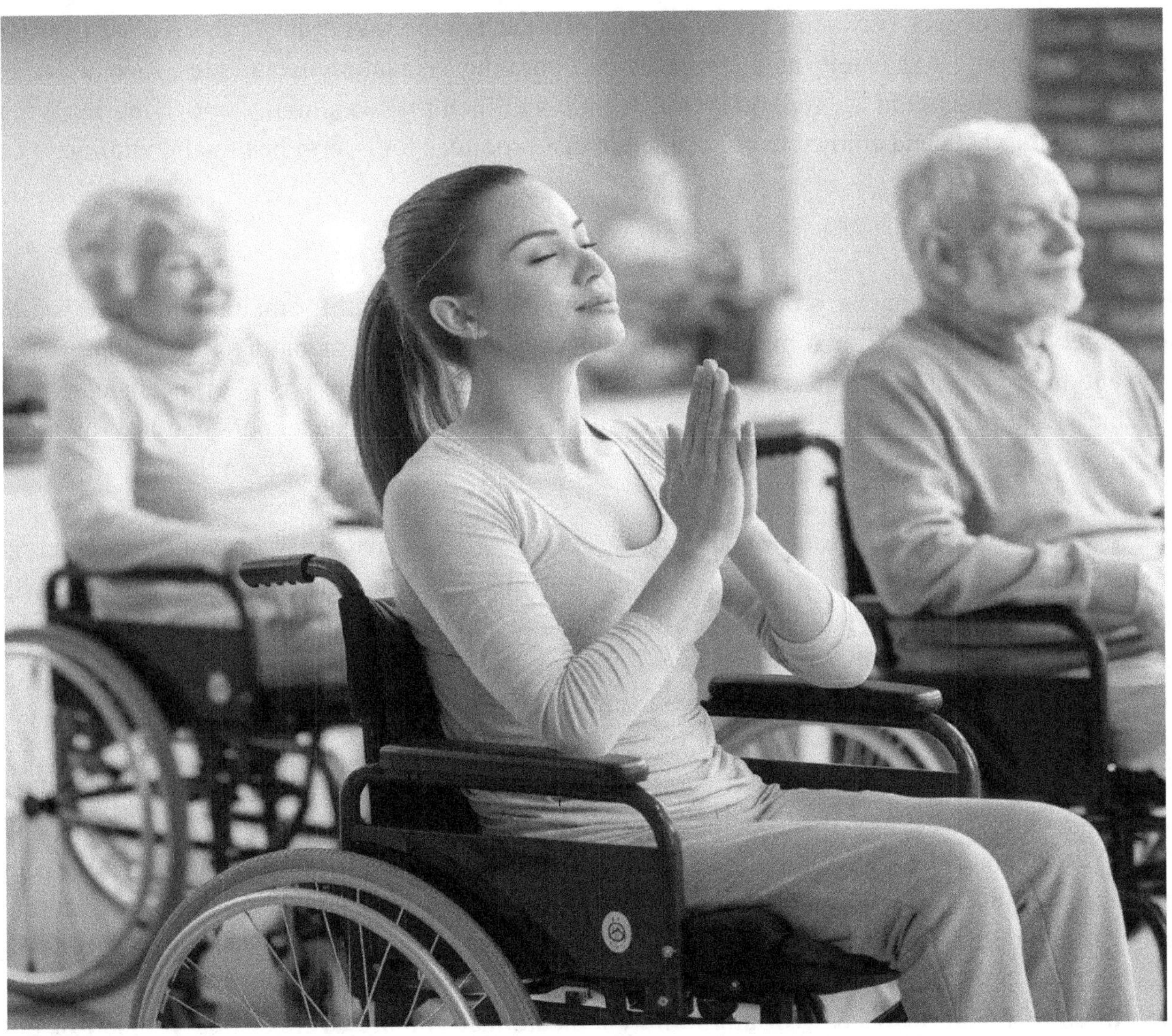

Start slowly and gradually increase the intensity and duration of your sessions. Beginning with shorter sessions allows your body to acclimate to the new movements and routines without becoming overwhelmed. As your strength and flexibility improve, you can extend the length of your practice and incorporate more challenging exercises. Patience and consistency are key to building a sustainable and safe yoga practice over time.

Use proper alignment and technique to maximize the benefits of each exercise while minimizing the risk of injury. Focus on maintaining a straight spine, engaging your core muscles, and performing movements with controlled, deliberate motions. Avoid rushing through poses; instead, take the time to move thoughtfully and with intention. Proper technique enhances the effectiveness of your practice and helps prevent common mistakes that can lead to discomfort or injury.

Try to always corporate regular breaks and rest periods into your yoga sessions. Allowing your body time to recover between exercises helps prevent fatigue and reduces the risk of overuse injuries. Hydrate adequately and consider incorporating relaxation techniques such as deep breathing or meditation to support your overall well-being. Recognizing and honoring your limits fosters a safe and enjoyable yoga practice that promotes long-term health and vitality.

Recognizing Warning Signs

Being aware of warning signs during your yoga practice is essential for maintaining your health and safety. Certain symptoms may indicate that you need to stop or modify your exercises to prevent injury or adverse effects. Common warning signs include sharp or persistent pain, dizziness, shortness of breath, nausea, or excessive fatigue. If you experience any of these symptoms, it is important to cease the activity immediately and assess your condition.

Sharp or persistent pain during or after yoga exercises can signal that you are overextending yourself or performing a movement incorrectly. Unlike the mild discomfort associated with stretching muscles, sharp pain is a clear indicator that something is wrong. Pay attention to the location and intensity of the pain, and avoid pushing through it. Instead, adjust the exercise to a less intense version or try a different movement that does not cause discomfort.

Dizziness or lightheadedness can occur if you move too quickly or fail to maintain proper breathing during your practice. Ensure that you are performing exercises at a steady pace and taking deep, controlled breaths to maintain adequate oxygen flow. If you feel dizzy, pause your practice, sit quietly, and breathe deeply until the sensation passes. Avoid sudden movements that can disrupt your balance and contribute to feelings of dizziness.

Shortness of breath or excessive fatigue may indicate that you are overexerting yourself or not pacing your exercises appropriately. Chair yoga should enhance your energy levels, not deplete them. Monitor your breathing and ensure that you are not holding your breath during movements. Incorporate rest periods as needed and adjust the intensity of your exercises to match your current energy levels and stamina.

Be mindful of any unusual symptoms such as chest pain, irregular heartbeats, or swelling in your limbs. These could be signs of more serious underlying health issues that require immediate medical attention. In such cases, stop your practice and seek professional medical advice promptly. Recognizing and responding to warning signs helps you maintain a safe and beneficial chair yoga practice, supporting your overall health and well-being.

When to Consult a Healthcare Professional

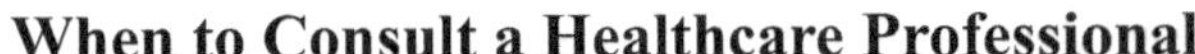

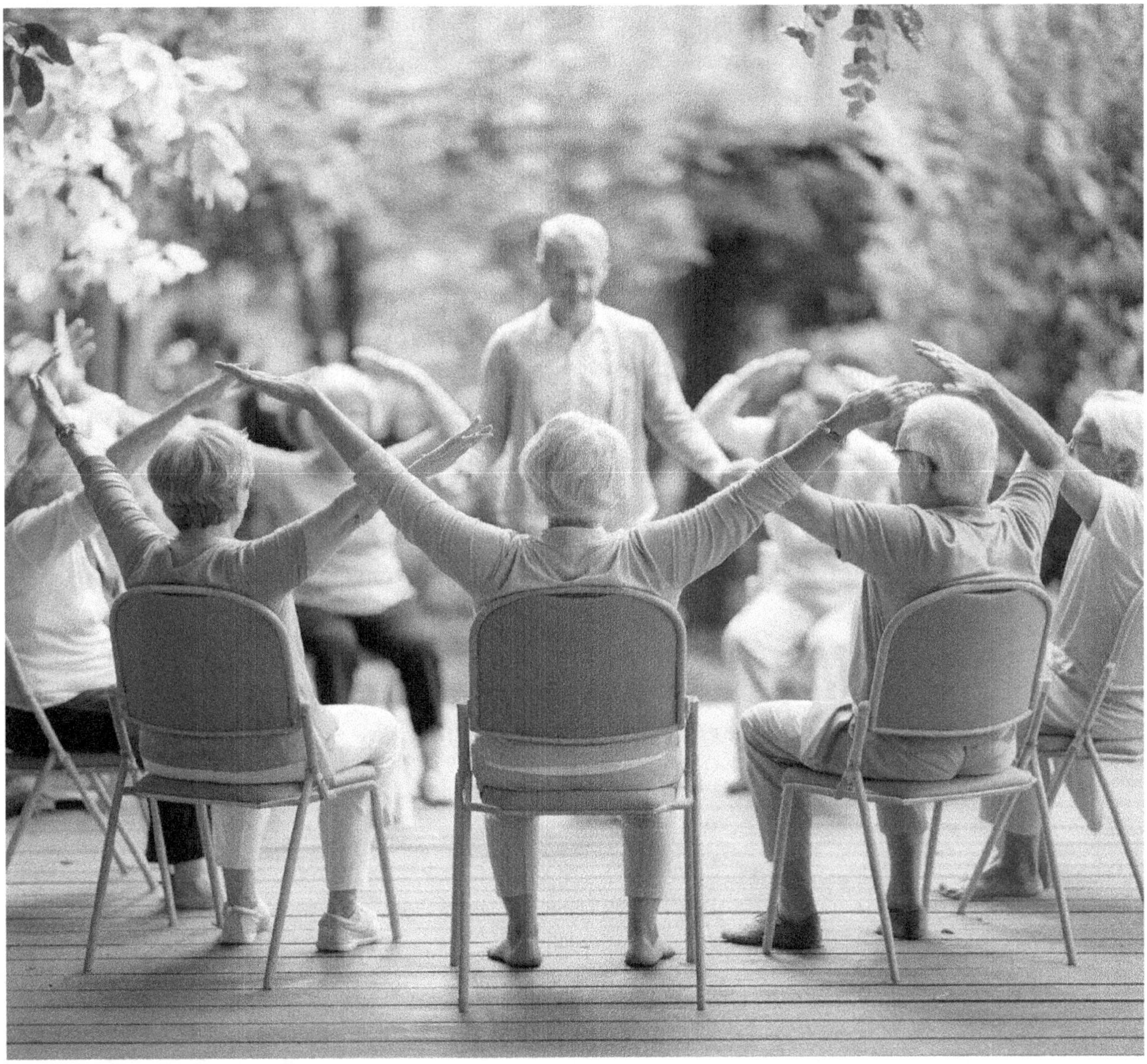

Before embarking on a chair yoga journey, it is advisable to consult with a healthcare professional, especially if you have pre-existing health conditions or concerns. A healthcare provider can offer personalized advice based on your medical history, current health status, and specific needs. This consultation ensures that chair yoga is a safe and appropriate form of exercise for you, and helps identify any modifications or precautions you should take during your practice.

Regular check-ins with your healthcare provider are beneficial, particularly if you experience changes in your health or new symptoms while practicing chair yoga. These updates allow your provider to monitor your progress and make necessary adjustments to your exercise regimen. Open communication with your healthcare team ensures that your yoga practice continues to support your health goals safely and effectively.

Certain medical conditions may require specific modifications to your chair yoga practice. For example, individuals with osteoporosis may need to avoid certain poses that place excessive stress on the spine, while those with arthritis may benefit from gentle, low-impact movements that reduce joint stiffness. Your healthcare provider can guide you in selecting appropriate exercises and advise on any movements to avoid, ensuring that your practice aligns with your health needs.

In addition to medical conditions, your healthcare provider can offer valuable insights into the intensity and frequency of your yoga sessions. They can help you determine the optimal duration of your practice and recommend how often you should engage in chair yoga to achieve the best results without overexerting yourself. This personalized approach enhances the effectiveness of your practice and supports your long-term health and wellness.

If you encounter any health issues or complications during your chair yoga practice, consulting with a healthcare professional is essential. Whether it's persistent pain, unexpected fatigue, or other concerning symptoms, seeking medical advice promptly can prevent minor issues from escalating into more serious problems. Prioritizing your health by maintaining regular communication with your healthcare provider ensures that your chair yoga practice remains a safe and beneficial component of your overall wellness routine.

Chapter 3

UNDERSTANDING YOUR BODY

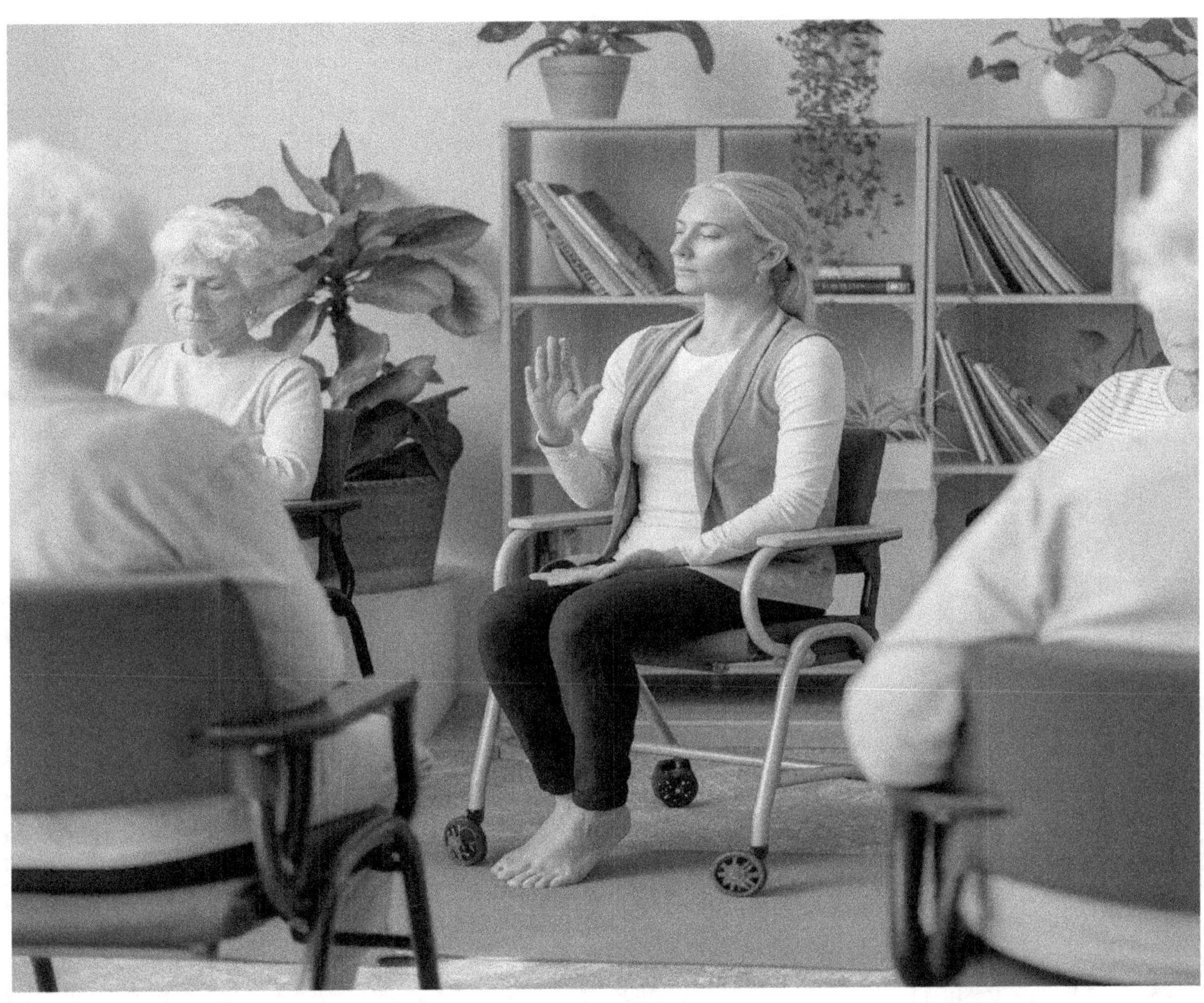

In this chapter , I will guide you through the essential fundamentals that form the backbone of a successful stretching and fitness journey. I begin by exploring the intricate anatomy of the muscles, joints, and connective tissues, providing you with a clear picture of how your body moves and functions. Understanding these components is crucial, especially for seniors, as it helps in identifying your body's unique strengths and areas that may require extra attention. I emphasize the importance of recognizing personal limitations and listening to your body's signals to prevent injuries and ensure a safe practice. Additionally, I introduce the concept of body awareness, which enhances your ability to perform exercises with proper alignment and technique, maximizing their effectiveness. By the end of this chapter, you will have a deeper appreciation of your physical self, empowering you to make informed decisions about your stretching routines and set realistic, achievable fitness goals. This foundational knowledge not only supports your immediate health and flexibility improvements but also fosters long-term wellness and mobility, ensuring that your fitness journey is both enjoyable and sustainable.

The Aging Body and Flexibility

How Aging Affects Mobility

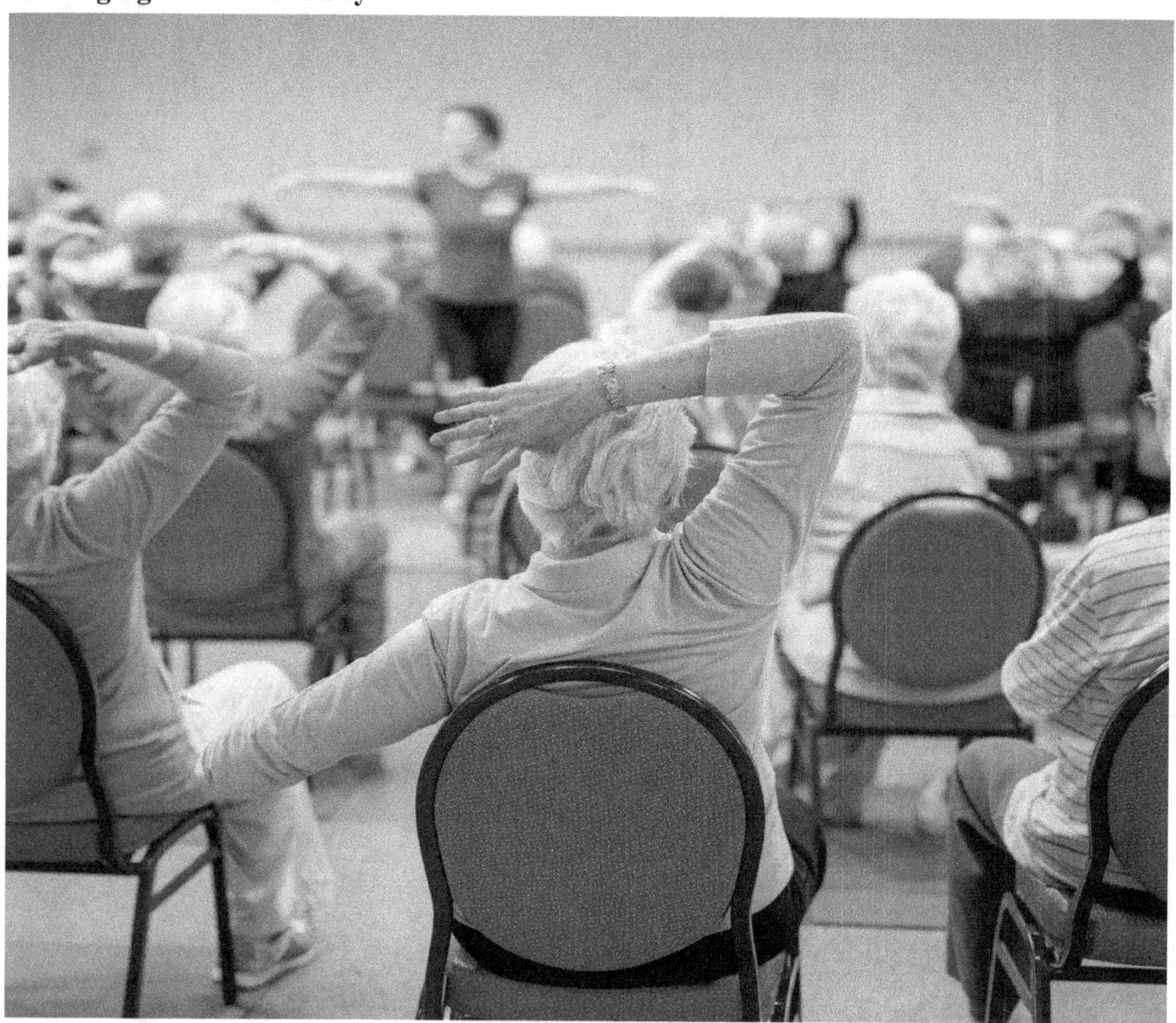

As we age, our bodies undergo a myriad of changes that can significantly impact mobility. The natural aging process leads to a gradual loss of muscle mass and bone density, which can make movement more challenging and increase the risk of fractures. Additionally, the cartilage that cushions our joints begins to wear down, resulting in stiffness and discomfort. These physiological changes can limit our range of motion, making everyday activities feel more strenuous. Understanding these changes is crucial for seniors who wish to maintain an active lifestyle through practices like chair yoga.

Moreover, the decrease in flexibility often accompanies other age-related issues such as decreased circulation and slower metabolism. Reduced blood flow can lead to muscle cramps and a general sense of sluggishness, further hindering mobility. The nervous system also experiences a decline in efficiency, affecting coordination and balance. These factors collectively contribute to a diminished ability to move freely and comfortably, highlighting the importance of targeted exercises to combat these challenges.

Despite these changes, it's important to recognize that mobility can still be improved with consistent effort and the right approach. Engaging in regular physical activity, particularly low-impact exercises like chair yoga, can help mitigate the effects of aging on the body. By focusing on gentle stretching and strengthening, seniors can maintain and even enhance their mobility, allowing them to enjoy a higher quality of life. Embracing these practices can make a significant difference in daily functioning and overall well-being.

Furthermore, maintaining mobility is not just about physical health; it also plays a vital role in mental and emotional well-being. Being able to move freely and perform daily tasks independently fosters a sense of autonomy and self-esteem. It reduces feelings of dependency and helplessness, which are common among seniors experiencing mobility issues. By actively working to preserve mobility, individuals can maintain a more positive outlook and remain engaged in their communities and personal interests.

Aging inevitably affects mobility, but it does not spell the end of an active and fulfilling life. Understanding the specific ways in which mobility is impacted allows seniors to take proactive steps to preserve and enhance their movement capabilities. Chair yoga offers a safe and effective means to address these challenges, providing a pathway to sustained mobility and improved quality of life.

Benefits of Maintaining Flexibility

Maintaining flexibility as we age offers numerous benefits that extend beyond physical health. Flexible muscles and joints contribute to better posture, which can alleviate common aches and pains associated with aging, such as back and neck discomfort. Improved posture not only enhances physical appearance but also supports the skeletal structure, reducing the likelihood of developing chronic pain conditions. By incorporating flexibility exercises into daily routines, seniors can experience significant relief from discomfort and enhance their overall physical comfort.

Flexibility also plays a crucial role in enhancing balance and stability. As muscles remain supple and joints retain their range of motion, the body is better equipped to maintain balance, reducing the risk of falls—a common and serious concern among older adults. Improved balance contributes to greater confidence in movement, encouraging seniors to remain active and independent. This increased confidence can lead to a more active lifestyle, further promoting physical health and mobility.

Moreover, flexibility exercises can enhance circulation and promote better blood flow throughout the body. Increased circulation aids in the delivery of oxygen and essential nutrients to muscles and tissues, facilitating quicker recovery from physical exertion and reducing the risk of injuries. Enhanced blood flow also supports the removal of metabolic waste products, which can decrease inflammation and muscle soreness. These circulatory benefits contribute to overall vitality and energy levels, making daily activities feel less taxing.

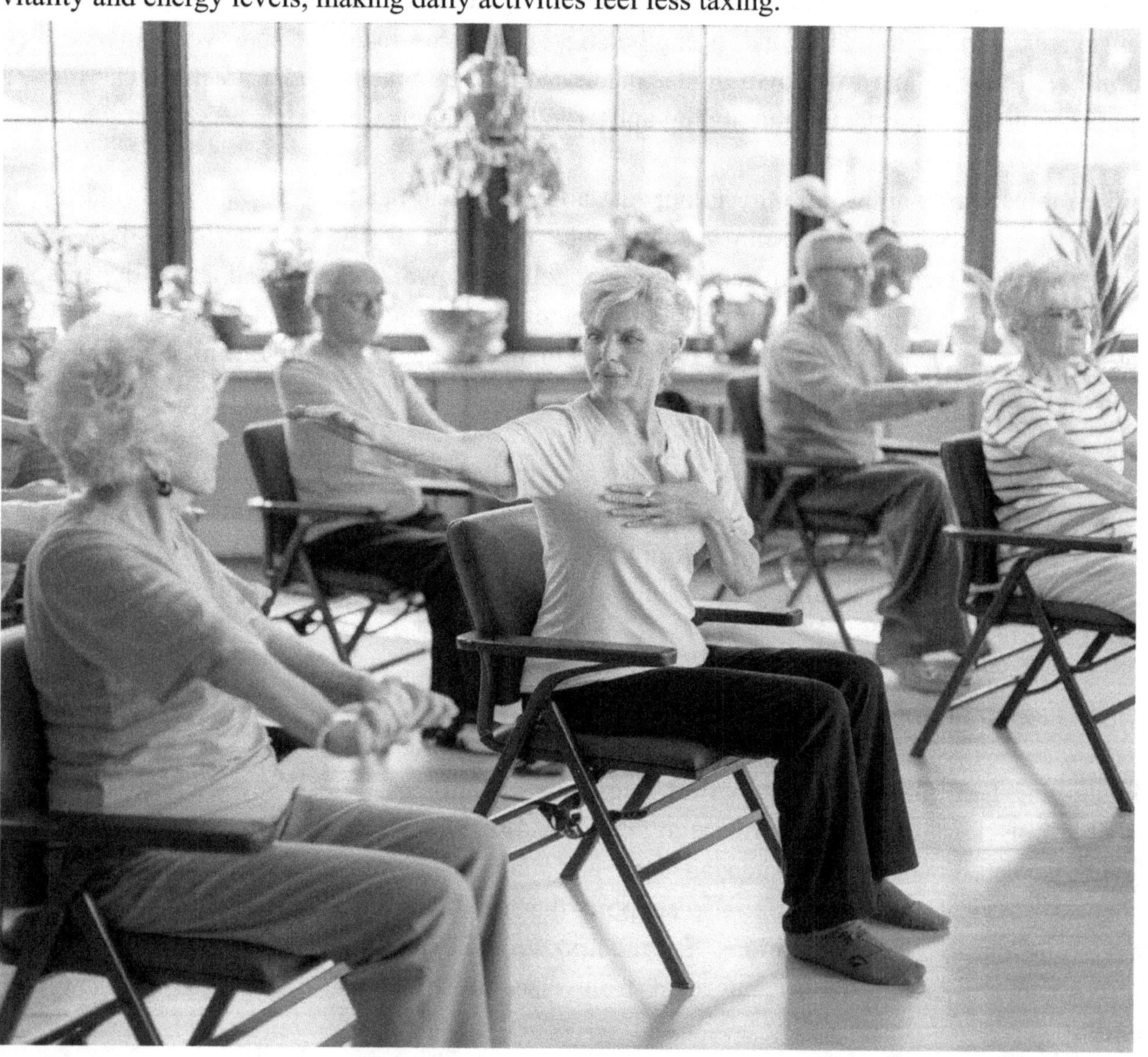

In addition to physical benefits, maintaining flexibility has positive effects on mental and emotional well-being. Engaging in regular stretching and movement can reduce stress and promote relaxation, contributing to a calmer and more focused mind. The rhythmic nature of flexibility exercises can also serve as a form of meditation, providing a mental break from the stresses of daily life. This holistic approach to health underscores the interconnectedness of the body and mind, highlighting the comprehensive benefits of maintaining flexibility.

Flexibility enhances the ability to perform everyday tasks with ease and efficiency. From reaching for items on high shelves to bending down to tie shoes, a flexible body can adapt to various movements without strain or discomfort. This increased ease in performing daily activities fosters a greater sense of independence and self-sufficiency, essential components of a fulfilling and dignified life in later years. By prioritizing flexibility, seniors can maintain their autonomy and enjoy a higher quality of life.

Adapting Exercises to Your Body

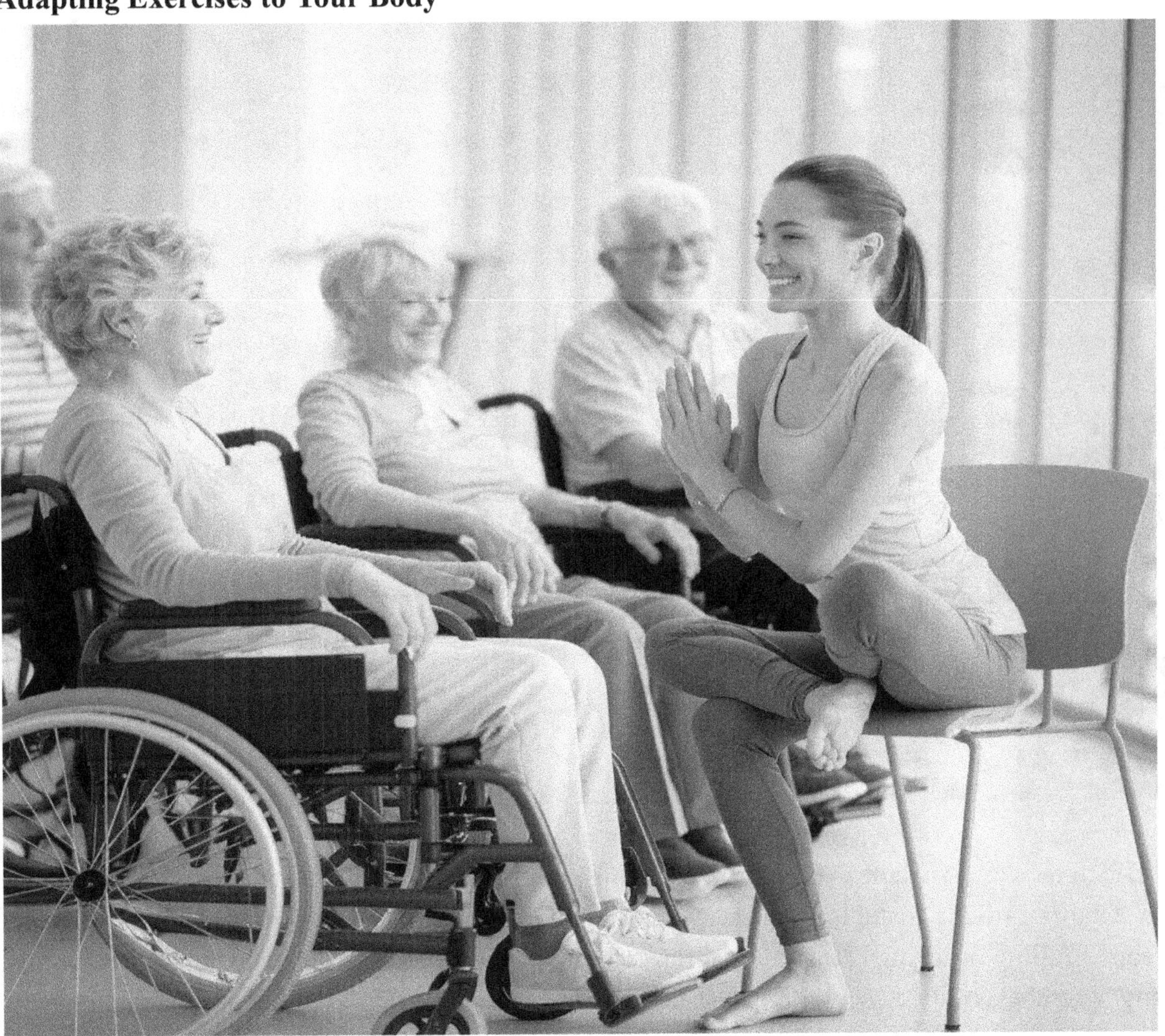

Adapting yoga exercises to suit individual needs is essential for ensuring safety and maximizing benefits, especially for seniors over 70. Each person's body is unique, with varying levels of flexibility, strength, and mobility. By customizing exercises to accommodate these differences, seniors can engage in yoga practices that are both effective and comfortable. This personalized approach helps prevent injuries and ensures that each session contributes positively to overall health and well-being.

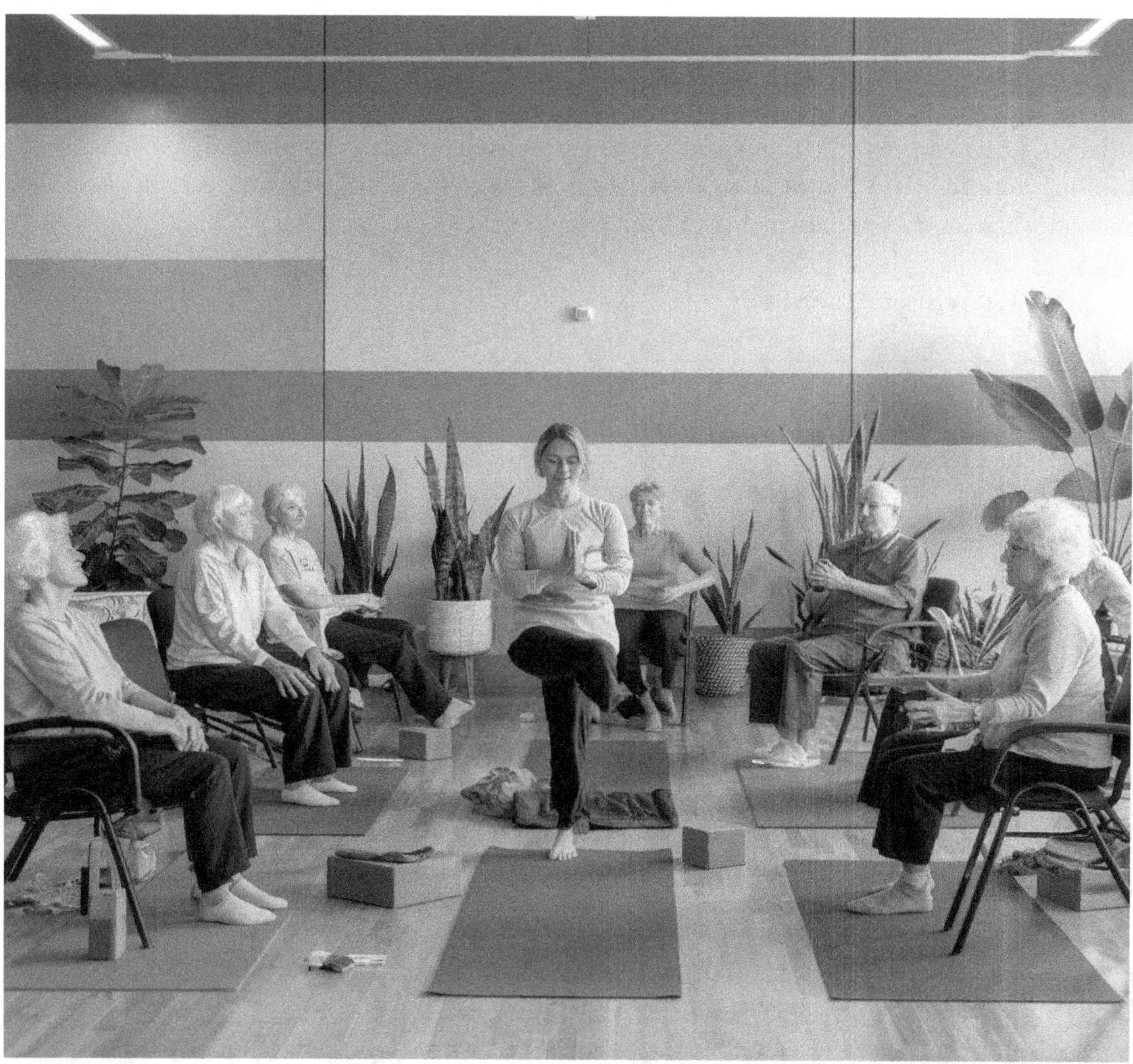

One effective way to adapt exercises is by using props such as chairs, cushions, and resistance bands. Chairs provide a stable support system, allowing seniors to perform movements without the fear of falling or losing balance. Cushions can offer additional comfort and support for joints, making stretches more accessible. Resistance bands can add an extra layer of challenge to strength-building exercises, enabling gradual progression as strength improves. These tools enhance the adaptability of yoga routines, making them suitable for a wide range of physical abilities.

Modifying poses is another crucial aspect of adapting exercises. Simple adjustments, such as reducing the range of motion or altering the position of limbs, can make poses more manageable. For instance, a full forward bend can be modified by only reaching the arms halfway forward, reducing strain on the back and legs. Similarly, seated twists can be performed with a smaller twist angle, maintaining spinal alignment and minimizing discomfort. These modifications allow seniors to experience the benefits of yoga without overexerting themselves.

Listening to the body's signals is paramount when adapting exercises. It's important for seniors to pay attention to how their bodies feel during and after each movement. Discomfort or pain should be taken as a sign to ease off or adjust the exercise accordingly. Gentle stretching should never cause sharp pain; instead, it should create a mild tension that gradually releases. By being attuned to their bodies, seniors can make informed decisions about how to adapt their yoga practice to suit their current physical state.

Seeking guidance from a qualified instructor can greatly enhance the ability to adapt exercises effectively. Yoga instructors trained in chair yoga for seniors can provide valuable insights and personalized adjustments that align with individual needs and limitations. They can offer hands-on assistance and feedback, ensuring that each movement is performed correctly and safely. This professional support fosters a more effective and enjoyable yoga practice, empowering seniors to embrace yoga as a lifelong companion in their journey toward health and wellness.

Common Joint and Muscle Issues

Addressing Arthritis and Joint Pain

Arthritis is a prevalent condition among seniors, characterized by inflammation and pain in the joints. This condition can significantly impair mobility and reduce the quality of life. Chair yoga offers a gentle yet effective way to manage arthritis symptoms by promoting joint flexibility and reducing stiffness. Through carefully designed movements, seniors can engage their joints in a safe manner, alleviating discomfort and enhancing overall joint function.

One of the primary benefits of chair yoga for arthritis sufferers is the reduction of inflammation. Regular stretching and movement help increase blood flow to the affected joints, facilitating the removal of inflammatory substances and promoting healing. Additionally, yoga encourages the release of endorphins, the body's natural painkillers, which can help manage chronic pain associated with arthritis. These physiological responses contribute to a decrease in joint swelling and an overall improvement in joint health.

Strengthening the muscles around arthritic joints is another critical aspect of managing joint pain. Strong muscles provide better support and stability for the joints, reducing the strain and preventing further deterioration. Chair yoga includes strength-building exercises that target key muscle groups without placing excessive pressure on the joints. This balanced approach helps maintain muscle mass and joint integrity, essential for long-term joint health and pain management.

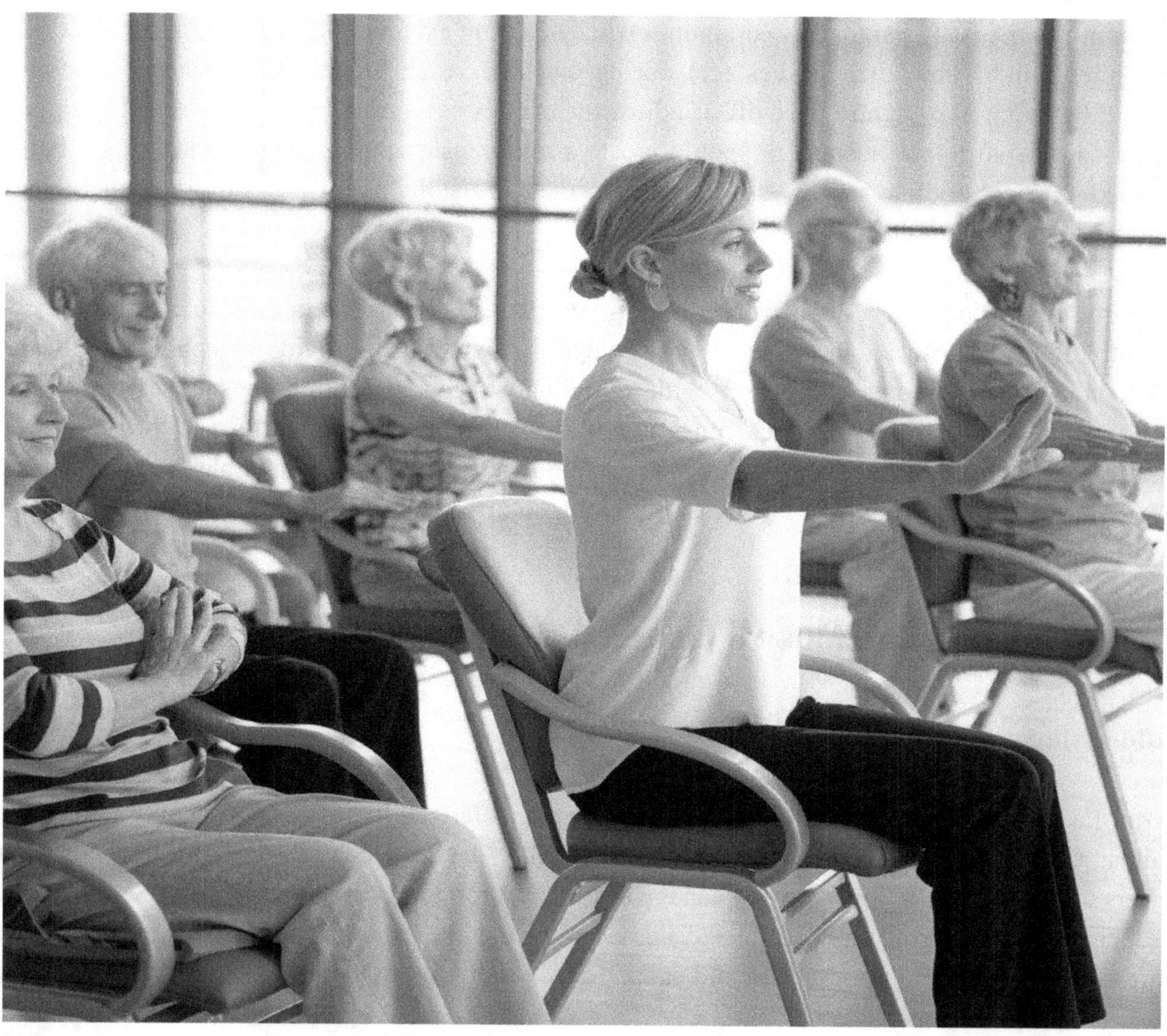

Flexibility exercises within chair yoga routines also play a significant role in addressing arthritis. Gentle stretching helps maintain and improve the range of motion in affected joints, preventing the development of contractures and maintaining functional mobility. Regular flexibility training ensures that joints remain supple and can move smoothly, reducing the likelihood of painful stiffness and enhancing the ease of daily movements. This sustained flexibility contributes to a more active and less painful lifestyle.

Chair yoga fosters a holistic approach to arthritis management by integrating physical movement with mental well-being. Practices such as deep breathing and meditation reduce stress, which can exacerbate pain perception. By promoting relaxation and mental clarity, yoga helps seniors cope with the emotional challenges of living with arthritis. This comprehensive approach not only addresses the physical symptoms but also supports emotional resilience, enabling seniors to navigate arthritis with greater ease and confidence.

Managing Muscle Stiffness

Muscle stiffness is a common issue faced by seniors, often resulting from prolonged periods of inactivity, aging, or underlying health conditions. Stiff muscles can limit mobility, reduce flexibility, and cause significant discomfort, making daily activities more challenging. Chair yoga offers an effective solution for managing muscle stiffness by incorporating gentle stretches and movements that target key muscle groups, enhancing flexibility and promoting muscle relaxation.

One of the key strategies in chair yoga for alleviating muscle stiffness is regular stretching. Stretching helps elongate tight muscles, reducing tension and improving overall flexibility. By engaging in consistent stretching routines, seniors can gradually increase the suppleness of their muscles, making movements smoother and less painful. This regularity not only alleviates current stiffness but also prevents the recurrence of tightness, fostering long-term muscle health.

In addition to stretching, chair yoga incorporates dynamic movements that encourage muscle activation and circulation. Gentle, controlled movements help stimulate blood flow to the muscles, delivering essential nutrients and oxygen that aid in muscle recovery and reduce stiffness. Enhanced circulation also facilitates the removal of metabolic waste products, which can accumulate and contribute to muscle soreness and tightness. These benefits collectively enhance muscle function and reduce the incidence of stiffness.

Strengthening exercises within chair yoga routines also play a vital role in managing muscle stiffness. Strengthening muscles increases their endurance and resilience, making them less prone to fatigue and tightness. By focusing on building muscle strength through targeted exercises, seniors can support their muscles more effectively, reducing the likelihood of stiffness caused by overuse or strain. Stronger muscles also contribute to better posture and alignment, further decreasing the risk of muscle-related discomfort.

Incorporating relaxation techniques into chair yoga sessions aids in managing muscle stiffness. Practices such as deep breathing and guided relaxation help calm the nervous system, reducing muscle tension and promoting a state of relaxation. This mental relaxation complements the physical stretching and strengthening, creating a synergistic effect that enhances overall muscle flexibility and comfort. By addressing both the physical and mental aspects of muscle stiffness, chair yoga provides a comprehensive approach to maintaining muscle health and reducing stiffness.

Preventing Injuries

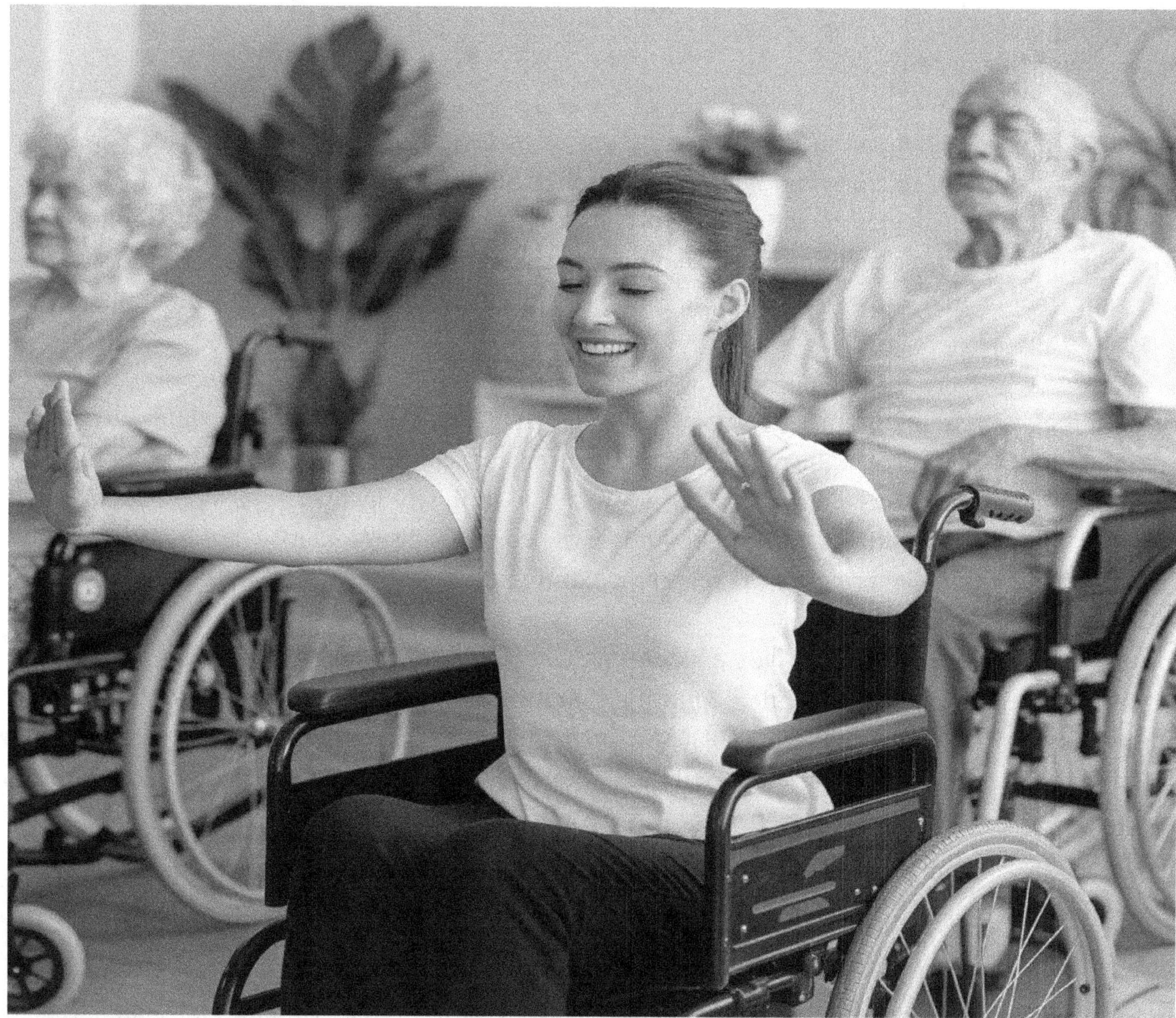

Preventing injuries is paramount for seniors engaging in any form of physical activity, including chair yoga. As the body ages, tissues become more fragile, and the risk of injury increases. Chair yoga, when performed correctly and with appropriate modifications, offers a safe way to enhance strength, flexibility, and balance without placing undue stress on the body. By understanding and implementing injury prevention strategies, seniors can enjoy the benefits of yoga while minimizing the risk of harm.

One fundamental aspect of injury prevention in chair yoga is proper alignment. Ensuring that each movement is performed with correct posture and alignment reduces the strain on muscles and joints, preventing overextension and undue pressure. Instructors and participants alike should focus on maintaining a neutral spine, aligning the knees over the ankles, and keeping the shoulders relaxed and away from the ears. This attention to alignment fosters safe and effective practice, safeguarding against potential injuries.

Another critical strategy is the gradual progression of exercises. Seniors should start with basic movements and slowly increase the intensity and complexity of their routines as their strength and flexibility improve. Rushing into advanced poses or pushing beyond comfortable limits can lead to strains, sprains, and other injuries. By adhering to a steady and manageable pace, seniors can build their capabilities safely, ensuring that their bodies are adequately prepared for each new challenge.

Listening to the body is also essential for injury prevention. Seniors should pay close attention to how their bodies respond during yoga sessions, recognizing the difference between normal discomfort and pain that signals potential injury. If a movement causes sharp pain, dizziness, or excessive fatigue, it should be stopped immediately. Adjustments or alternative exercises should be sought to accommodate individual limitations, ensuring that yoga remains a safe and enjoyable practice.

Be informed that incorporating warm-up and cool-down routines into each chair yoga session can significantly reduce the risk of injury. Warm-ups prepare the muscles and joints for activity by increasing blood flow and enhancing flexibility, making them less susceptible to strains. Cool-downs, on the other hand, help the body transition back to a state of rest, preventing muscle stiffness and promoting recovery. These preparatory and concluding practices bookend each yoga session with layers of protection, fostering a safer exercise environment for seniors.

Listening to Your Body

Mind-Body Connection

The mind-body connection is a fundamental principle in yoga, emphasizing the interplay between mental and physical states. For seniors, cultivating this connection can lead to profound improvements in overall well-being. By focusing on the sensations within their bodies and the rhythms of their breath, seniors can enhance their awareness and foster a deeper sense of presence. This heightened awareness not only improves the effectiveness of yoga practices but also contributes to a more mindful and balanced life.

Engaging the mind-body connection involves paying close attention to how each movement feels, rather than merely going through the motions. Seniors are encouraged to notice the subtle changes in muscle tension, joint movement, and breathing patterns. This attentiveness allows them to respond to their bodies' needs, making adjustments as necessary to maintain comfort and safety. By tuning into these internal signals, seniors can practice yoga in a way that honors their physical limitations and promotes harmony between mind and body.

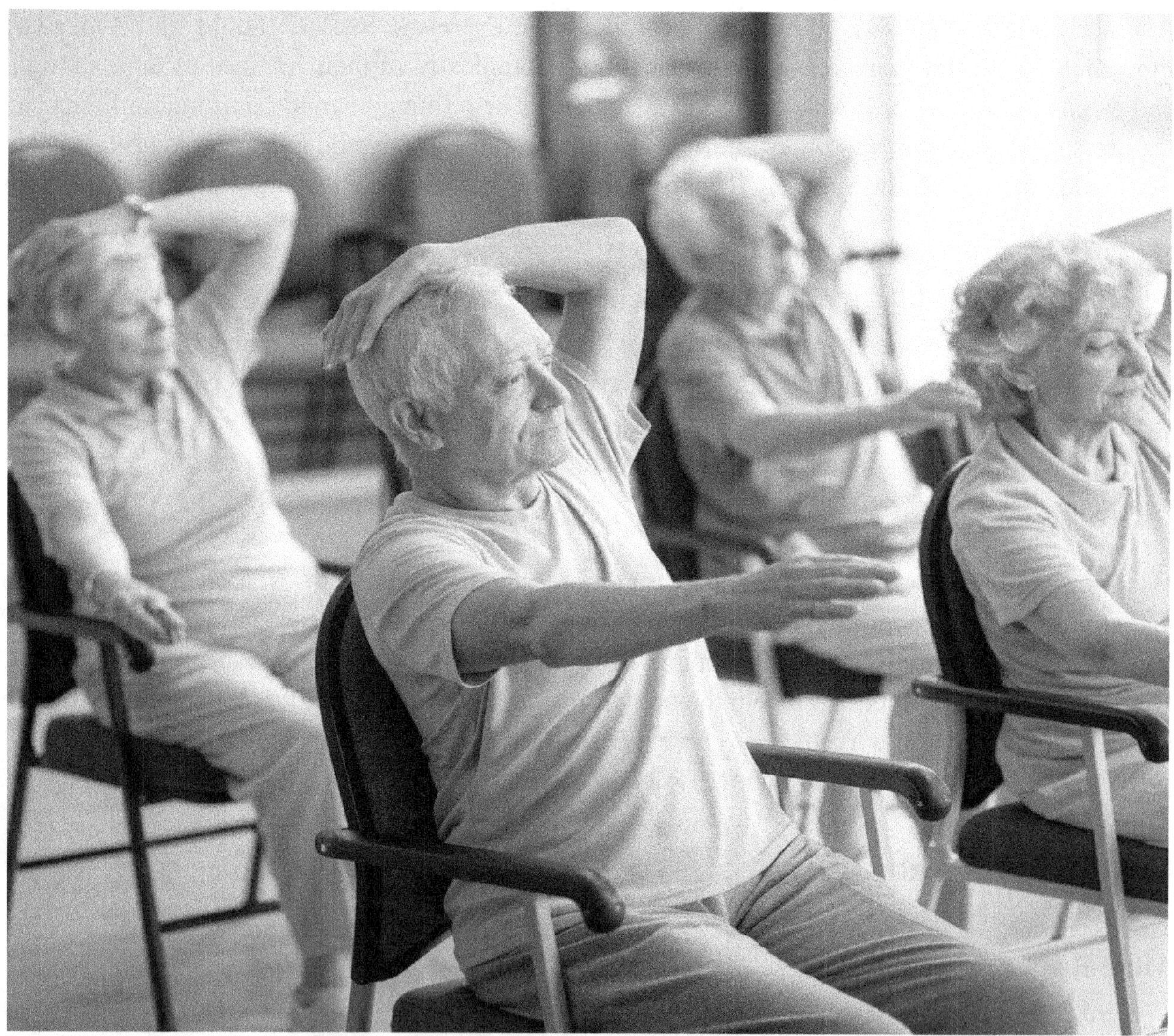

Moreover, the mind-body connection enhances mental clarity and emotional resilience. Practices such as deep breathing and meditation, integral to chair yoga, help calm the mind and reduce stress. This mental calmness can lead to improved focus and concentration, making it easier to perform yoga movements with intention and precision. Additionally, the sense of accomplishment that comes from mindful movement can boost self-esteem and foster a positive outlook, contributing to overall emotional well-being.

Another benefit of the mind-body connection is its role in pain management. By becoming more attuned to their bodies, seniors can better understand the sources of their discomfort and address them proactively. Mindfulness techniques can help reframe the perception of pain, reducing its intensity and impact on daily life. This approach empowers seniors to take control of their pain, utilizing yoga as a tool for both physical relief and mental empowerment.

Nurturing the mind-body connection through chair yoga encourages a holistic approach to health. It reinforces the idea that physical health is deeply intertwined with mental and emotional states, promoting a comprehensive view of well-being. This integrated perspective motivates seniors to engage in practices that support all aspects of their health, leading to a more balanced and fulfilling life. By fostering this connection, chair yoga becomes more than just a physical exercise—it becomes a pathway to holistic wellness.

Modifying Poses for Comfort

Modifying yoga poses to suit individual comfort levels is essential for creating a safe and enjoyable practice, particularly for seniors. Each person's body has unique strengths, limitations, and areas of sensitivity, making it important to tailor exercises accordingly. Chair yoga provides the flexibility to adjust poses, ensuring that seniors can engage in yoga without experiencing discomfort or strain. These modifications not only enhance safety but also make yoga more accessible and sustainable for long-term practice.

One common modification involves using props such as cushions, blankets, and resistance bands to support the body during poses. For example, placing a cushion behind the lower back can provide additional support during seated twists, reducing strain on the spine. Similarly, using a resistance band for arm stretches can help seniors perform movements with greater control and less effort. These supportive tools make poses more comfortable and attainable, allowing seniors to experience the benefits of yoga without pushing beyond their limits.

Another key modification is adjusting the range of motion in each pose. Instead of striving for full extension or deep bends, seniors can perform movements within a comfortable and manageable range. For instance, a gentle forward bend can be achieved by only leaning slightly forward, rather than reaching all the way down to the toes. This approach prevents overextension and reduces the risk of injury, making yoga a more pleasurable and less intimidating experience.

Additionally, changing the angle or orientation of the body can help accommodate specific physical conditions. For example, if a senior experiences knee pain, they can adjust the angle of their legs during seated stretches to minimize discomfort. Alternatively, leaning slightly back during a twist can alleviate pressure on the lower back. These subtle adjustments ensure that each pose aligns with the individual's physical needs, promoting comfort and effectiveness in their yoga practice.

Incorporating rest breaks and pauses between poses is an important modification for maintaining comfort. Seniors should feel empowered to take short breaks whenever needed, allowing their bodies to recover and preventing fatigue. These pauses can be used to focus on breathing, reassess comfort levels, and prepare for the next movement. By integrating rest periods, chair yoga becomes a more sustainable and enjoyable practice, enabling seniors to engage in yoga consistently without overexertion.

Importance of Rest and Recovery

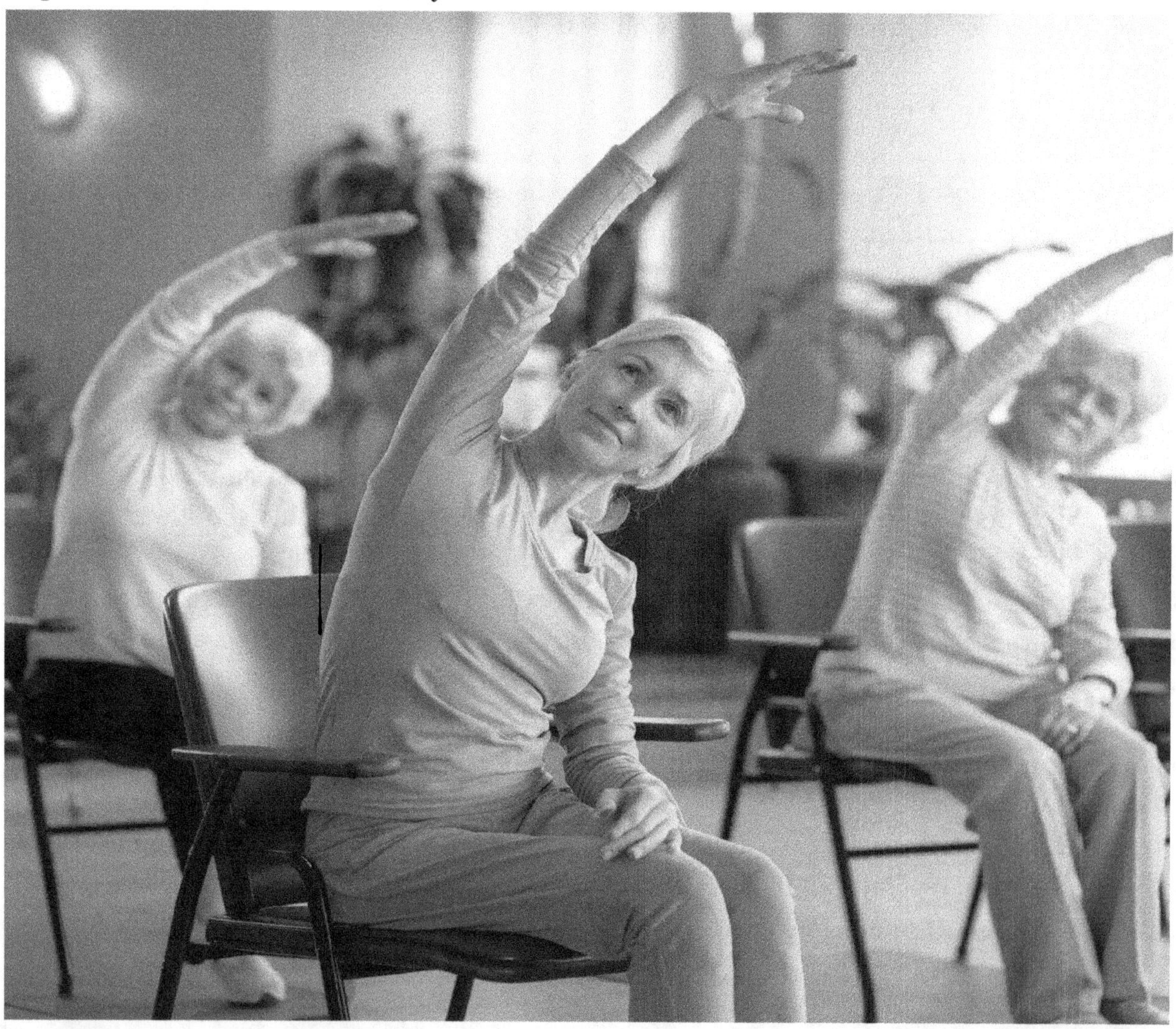

Rest and recovery are integral components of any exercise regimen, including chair yoga. For seniors, the significance of adequate rest cannot be overstated, as the body's ability to heal and rejuvenate diminishes with age. Incorporating rest periods into a yoga routine allows the muscles and joints to recover from exertion, preventing overuse injuries and promoting long-term health. Understanding the balance between activity and rest is essential for maintaining a sustainable and beneficial yoga practice.

During rest periods, the body undergoes vital repair processes that strengthen muscles and restore energy levels. After engaging in physical activity, muscles experience tiny tears that need time to heal and rebuild. This healing process not only increases muscle strength but also enhances flexibility and endurance. Without sufficient rest, these repair mechanisms are compromised, leading to muscle fatigue, soreness, and an increased risk of injury. Therefore, allowing time for recovery is crucial for maximizing the benefits of yoga.

Mental recovery is equally important, especially for seniors who may experience increased stress and fatigue. Rest periods provide an opportunity to relax the mind, reducing mental strain and promoting a sense of calm. Practices such as deep breathing and meditation during rest breaks can enhance mental clarity and emotional stability, contributing to overall well-being. This mental relaxation complements the physical benefits of yoga, fostering a holistic approach to health.

Incorporating restorative poses into the yoga routine can enhance the benefits of rest and recovery. Gentle stretches and supported poses, such as seated forward bends or supported twists, allow the body to relax deeply while still engaging in beneficial movement. These restorative practices help alleviate muscle tension, improve circulation, and promote relaxation, facilitating a more effective recovery process. By integrating restorative elements, chair yoga sessions become more balanced and supportive of the body's natural healing processes.

Recognizing the signs of fatigue and respecting the body's need for rest are essential for maintaining a healthy yoga practice. Seniors should listen to their bodies, acknowledging when they need to slow down or take a break. Pushing through excessive fatigue can lead to burnout and diminish the overall enjoyment of yoga. By prioritizing rest and recovery, seniors can engage in yoga with greater consistency and joy, ensuring that their practice remains a source of health and happiness throughout their lives.

Chapter 4

BREATHING TECHNIQUES AND MEDITATION

In this chapter, I delve into the transformative power of breathing techniques and meditation, essential components of chair yoga that can profoundly enhance the well-being of seniors over 70. Having witnessed firsthand the remarkable benefits these practices offer, I am passionate about guiding you through simple yet effective methods to improve your respiratory health, reduce stress, and cultivate a sense of inner peace. I will explore various breathing exercises tailored to your unique needs, ensuring they are both accessible and impactful. Additionally, I will introduce meditation practices that promote mental clarity and emotional balance, helping you navigate the challenges of aging with grace and resilience. By integrating these techniques into your daily routine, you can experience heightened relaxation, increased energy levels, and a deeper connection between mind and body. My goal is to provide you with the tools and confidence to embrace these practices, empowering you to achieve a harmonious and fulfilling lifestyle through the mindful art of breathing and meditation.

Breathing Exercises for Relaxation

Deep Breathing Techniques

Deep breathing is a foundational practice in yoga and meditation, especially beneficial for seniors seeking relaxation and stress relief. This technique involves taking slow, deliberate breaths that fully engage the lungs, allowing for maximum oxygen intake. By focusing on deep breaths, individuals can activate the parasympathetic nervous system, which helps to calm the mind and reduce anxiety. For seniors, deep breathing can alleviate feelings of tension and promote a sense of tranquility, making it easier to navigate daily stresses. Regular practice of deep breathing can also enhance respiratory function, contributing to overall physical well-being.

Diaphragmatic Breathing

Diaphragmatic breathing, also known as belly breathing, emphasizes the use of the diaphragm to take full breaths. This technique encourages the expansion of the abdomen rather than the chest, allowing for deeper inhalation and more efficient oxygen exchange. For seniors, diaphragmatic breathing can improve lung capacity and strengthen respiratory muscles, which may decline with age. Additionally, this type of breathing promotes relaxation by lowering heart rate and reducing blood pressure. Incorporating diaphragmatic breathing into daily routines can help seniors manage stress, enhance focus, and improve overall cardiovascular health.

Breath Awareness Practices

Breath awareness involves paying close attention to the natural rhythm of breathing without attempting to alter it. This mindful practice fosters a deeper connection between the mind and body, enhancing present-moment awareness. For seniors, practicing breath awareness can aid in reducing mental clutter and promoting mental clarity. By focusing on each breath, individuals can cultivate a sense of calm and improve their ability to concentrate. Breath awareness also serves as a gateway to more advanced meditation practices, laying the groundwork for sustained mental and emotional well-being.

Progressive Relaxation through Breathing

Progressive relaxation is a technique that combines deep breathing with the systematic relaxation of different muscle groups. By inhaling deeply and exhaling slowly, seniors can focus on releasing tension from specific areas of the body, such as the shoulders, neck, and legs. This method not only enhances physical relaxation but also promotes mental calmness. Progressive relaxation through breathing can be particularly beneficial for seniors dealing with chronic pain or muscle stiffness, as it helps to alleviate discomfort and improve overall mobility. Regular practice can lead to a more relaxed state of mind and a greater sense of physical ease.

Integrating Breathing Exercises into Daily Life

Integrating breathing exercises into daily routines ensures that the benefits of relaxation are consistently experienced. Seniors can incorporate deep breathing, diaphragmatic breathing, and breath awareness into various activities, such as during meals, while watching television, or before bedtime. Setting aside dedicated time each day for breathing exercises can help establish a habitual practice, reinforcing the positive effects on both mind and body. Additionally, using breathing techniques during moments of stress or anxiety can provide immediate relief and enhance emotional resilience. By making breathing exercises a regular part of their lives, seniors can maintain a state of relaxation and improve their overall quality of life.

Introduction to Meditation

Benefits of Meditation for Seniors

Meditation offers a multitude of benefits tailored to the unique needs of seniors. Regular meditation practice can significantly reduce stress, anxiety, and depression, fostering a sense of inner peace and emotional stability. For seniors, meditation can enhance cognitive function, improving memory, attention, and overall mental clarity. Additionally, meditation promotes physical health by lowering blood pressure, boosting the immune system, and reducing chronic pain. The holistic benefits of meditation contribute to a higher quality of life, enabling seniors to maintain both mental and physical well-being as they age gracefully.

Simple Meditation Practices

Starting a meditation practice does not require extensive experience or special equipment, making it accessible for seniors of all backgrounds. Simple meditation practices include seated meditation, where individuals focus on their breath or a chosen mantra, and guided imagery, which involves visualizing peaceful scenes or positive outcomes. Another approachable method is loving-kindness meditation, which cultivates feelings of compassion and goodwill towards oneself and others. These practices can be performed in short sessions, ranging from five to twenty minutes, allowing seniors to gradually build their meditation habits without feeling overwhelmed. The simplicity and adaptability of these techniques make meditation an ideal tool for enhancing daily well-being.

Incorporating Mindfulness into Daily Life

Mindfulness, the practice of being fully present and engaged in the current moment, can be seamlessly integrated into everyday activities. For seniors, incorporating mindfulness into daily life means paying attention to simple tasks such as eating, walking, or even gardening with heightened awareness and intention. This approach not only enhances the enjoyment of daily activities but also reduces stress and increases overall satisfaction. Mindfulness encourages seniors to live more fully, appreciating each moment and fostering a deeper connection with their surroundings. By weaving mindfulness into their routines, seniors can cultivate a more balanced and fulfilling life.

Creating a Meditation Space

Having a dedicated space for meditation can enhance the effectiveness of the practice. Seniors can create a serene and comfortable environment by choosing a quiet corner in their home, free from distractions and clutter. Adding elements such as cushions, soft lighting, and calming décor can make the space inviting and conducive to relaxation. Personalizing the meditation area with items that inspire tranquility, such as candles, plants, or meaningful artwork, can further enhance the meditative experience. A designated meditation space serves as a physical reminder to practice regularly, helping seniors establish a consistent and enjoyable meditation routine.

Overcoming Common Meditation Challenges

While meditation offers numerous benefits, some seniors may encounter challenges when starting their practice. Common obstacles include difficulty maintaining focus, physical discomfort, or skepticism about its effectiveness. To overcome these challenges, it is important to approach meditation with patience and compassion. Starting with shorter sessions and gradually increasing the duration can help build concentration skills without causing frustration. Using supportive props, such as cushions or chairs, can alleviate physical discomfort and make the practice more accessible. Additionally, seeking guidance from meditation instructors or joining group sessions can provide encouragement and enhance the overall experience. By addressing these challenges thoughtfully, seniors can successfully incorporate meditation into their lives and reap its full benefits.

Combining Breath and Movement

Synchronizing Breath with Poses

The harmonious coordination of breath and movement is a cornerstone of yoga practice, enhancing both the physical and mental benefits of each pose. For seniors practicing chair yoga, synchronizing breath with each movement ensures that exercises are performed mindfully and safely. Inhaling deeply as you prepare for a pose and exhaling as you move can create a rhythm that promotes fluidity and grace. This synchronization helps to maintain focus, prevent injury, and maximize the effectiveness of each exercise. By aligning breath with movement, seniors can experience a deeper sense of connection between their bodies and minds, enhancing the overall yoga practice.

Enhancing Focus and Concentration

Combining breath and movement not only improves physical performance but also sharpens mental focus and concentration. The intentional act of breathing in coordination with each movement requires attention and presence, training the mind to stay engaged in the moment. This heightened focus can translate to other areas of life, improving cognitive functions such as memory and problem-solving skills. For seniors, enhancing focus and concentration through synchronized breath and movement can lead to greater mental clarity and a more centered, calm state of being. This practice fosters a meditative state, allowing seniors to fully immerse themselves in the yoga experience and gain deeper mental benefits.

Creating a Meditative Practice

Integrating breath and movement into yoga routines transforms physical exercise into a meditative practice. Each coordinated breath and movement becomes an opportunity for mindfulness, allowing seniors to enter a state of calm and reflection. This meditative approach to yoga enhances the relaxation response, reducing stress and promoting emotional balance. By viewing each session as a moving meditation, seniors can cultivate a sense of inner peace and spiritual well-being. This holistic practice not only strengthens the body but also nurtures the mind and spirit, contributing to a comprehensive sense of wellness and fulfillment.

Flowing Through Poses with Breath

Flowing through poses with breath creates a seamless and continuous movement that enhances the overall yoga experience. For seniors, this fluidity ensures that transitions between poses are smooth and controlled, minimizing the risk of injury and maximizing the benefits of each exercise. Flowing with breath helps maintain momentum and energy, making the practice more engaging and enjoyable. This dynamic movement encourages flexibility and strength while promoting cardiovascular health through gentle, sustained activity. By embracing the flow of breath and movement, seniors can experience a more dynamic and invigorating yoga practice that supports both physical and mental vitality.

Deepening the Practice through Breath-Movement Integration

As seniors become more comfortable with synchronizing breath and movement, they can deepen their yoga practice by exploring more complex integrations. This might involve longer sequences of poses linked by breath or incorporating pauses for breath awareness between movements. Deepening the practice in this way enhances the meditative quality of yoga, allowing for greater introspection and self-awareness. It also fosters resilience and adaptability, as seniors learn to navigate the ebb and flow of each session with grace and mindfulness. By continually refining the integration of breath and movement, seniors can sustain a rich and rewarding yoga practice that evolves with their personal growth and wellness goals.

Chapter 5

WARM-UP ROUTINES

Warming up before engaging in any physical activity is essential, and chair yoga is no exception. For seniors, especially those over 70, a proper warm-up routine can enhance the effectiveness of the exercises, reduce the risk of injury, and prepare the body both physically and mentally for the session ahead. This chapter delves into three critical aspects of warm-up routines: Gentle Stretching Exercises, Preparing Your Body for Yoga, and Incorporating Mobility Drills. Each section provides comprehensive guidance to ensure that your warm-up is both safe and beneficial.

Gentle Stretching Exercises

Engaging in gentle stretching exercises is the cornerstone of an effective warm-up routine in chair yoga. These exercises are designed to gradually increase blood flow to the muscles, enhance flexibility, and prepare the body for more intensive movements. Starting with neck and shoulder stretches, seniors can alleviate tension that often accumulates in these areas due to prolonged sitting or inactivity. Simple movements, such as slowly tilting the head from side to side or rolling the shoulders forward and backward, can significantly improve range of motion and reduce stiffness.

Arm and wrist mobility exercises follow, focusing on enhancing the dexterity and strength of the upper limbs. These movements are particularly beneficial for seniors who may experience reduced hand strength or joint discomfort. Exercises like wrist circles, finger stretches, and gentle arm raises not only prepare the arms for yoga poses but also contribute to maintaining overall upper body health. By incorporating these stretches, individuals can perform daily activities with greater ease and comfort.

Lower body warm-ups are equally important, even when practicing yoga from a chair. These exercises target the legs, hips, and lower back, areas that are crucial for maintaining mobility and stability. Simple leg extensions, ankle rotations, and seated marches can activate the muscles and joints, setting the stage for more dynamic movements later in the session. These warm-ups help in preventing muscle cramps and ensuring that the lower body is adequately prepared for the upcoming exercises.

In addition to specific muscle groups, incorporating full-body stretches can provide a holistic approach to warming up. Gentle twists, side bends, and forward bends performed while seated can enhance overall flexibility and promote a sense of relaxation. These movements not only prepare the body but also calm the mind, creating a balanced state that is conducive to effective yoga practice. By addressing both the physical and mental aspects of warm-up, seniors can achieve a more fulfilling and enjoyable yoga experience.

Ultimately, gentle stretching exercises serve as a vital component of chair yoga, ensuring that each session begins with a prepared and receptive body. By systematically addressing key muscle groups and promoting overall flexibility, these stretches lay the foundation for a safe and effective yoga practice. Incorporating these exercises into your routine can lead to improved mobility, reduced discomfort, and a heightened sense of well-being.

Preparing Your Body for Yoga

Preparing the body for yoga involves more than just performing physical movements; it encompasses strategies to enhance overall readiness and ensure a productive session. Increasing blood flow is a fundamental aspect of preparation, as it ensures that muscles receive adequate oxygen and nutrients. Gentle movements, such as seated marches or light tapping of the legs, can stimulate circulation without causing strain. Enhanced blood flow not only warms the muscles but also contributes to mental alertness, setting a positive tone for the yoga practice.

Activating key muscle groups is another critical step in preparing for yoga. This involves engaging specific muscles that will be used during the session, thereby improving their responsiveness and reducing the risk of injury. For instance, activating the core muscles through gentle seated twists or engaging the back muscles with slight shoulder squeezes can create a stable foundation for various yoga poses. By consciously engaging these muscles, seniors can enhance their posture and maintain better alignment throughout the practice.

Reducing muscle tension is essential for a comfortable and effective yoga session. Prolonged periods of inactivity or stress can lead to muscle tightness, which may hinder movement and cause discomfort. Techniques such as deep breathing, progressive muscle relaxation, and gentle stretching can help alleviate tension and promote a state of relaxation. By addressing muscle tightness before beginning the yoga exercises, seniors can move more freely and enjoy a more seamless practice.

Mental preparation is equally important as physical readiness. Taking a few moments to center the mind through breathing exercises or brief meditation can enhance focus and concentration. This mental clarity not only improves the quality of the yoga practice but also fosters a sense of calm and well-being. By aligning the mind with the body, seniors can achieve a more harmonious and effective yoga experience, maximizing the benefits of each session.

Preparing the body for yoga involves a combination of increasing blood flow, activating key muscle groups, reducing muscle tension, and achieving mental clarity. These preparatory steps ensure that the body is adequately ready to engage in the yoga practice, enhancing both safety and effectiveness. By incorporating these strategies into the warm-up routine, seniors can create a conducive environment for a fulfilling and beneficial yoga session.

Incorporating Mobility Drills

Incorporating mobility drills into the warm-up routine is essential for enhancing the overall flexibility and range of motion, which are crucial for effective chair yoga practice. Ankle and foot movements play a significant role in maintaining balance and stability. Simple exercises such as ankle circles, toe taps, and heel lifts can improve circulation and flexibility in the lower extremities. These movements not only prepare the feet and ankles for seated yoga poses but also contribute to better posture and reduced strain on the lower back.

Spinal flexibility exercises are vital for maintaining a healthy and agile spine, especially in seniors who may experience age-related stiffness or discomfort. Gentle seated twists, side bends, and forward bends can enhance spinal mobility, allowing for more fluid and comfortable movements during yoga practice. These exercises help in maintaining the natural curvature of the spine, reducing the risk of back pain, and promoting a more relaxed and open posture.

Hip and knee mobilization exercises target the large joints that support the body's movements and stability. Engaging in gentle hip circles, knee extensions, and seated leg swings can enhance the flexibility and strength of these joints. Improved mobility in the hips and knees not only facilitates a wider range of yoga poses but also contributes to better overall mobility in daily activities. These exercises help in reducing stiffness, preventing joint pain, and ensuring that the lower body remains agile and responsive.

In addition to specific joint movements, incorporating dynamic mobility drills can further enhance the effectiveness of the warm-up routine. These drills involve continuous and controlled movements that mimic the actions performed during yoga practice. Examples include seated marches with arm swings, gentle seated jogging, and coordinated upper and lower body movements. These dynamic drills not only improve coordination and balance but also elevate the heart rate slightly, contributing to a more comprehensive warm-up.

Integrating mobility drills into the warm-up routine fosters a proactive approach to maintaining joint health and flexibility. Regular practice of these exercises can lead to long-term benefits, such as increased range of motion, reduced joint pain, and enhanced overall mobility. By making mobility drills a consistent part of the warm-up, seniors can ensure that their bodies remain flexible and resilient, capable of supporting an active and healthy lifestyle through chair yoga.

Chapter 6

STRENGTH TRAINING FOR SENIORS

As the author, I am passionate about empowering seniors to embrace strength training as a vital component of their overall health and wellness journey. In this chapter, I delve into the numerous benefits that strength training offers for individuals over 70, including enhanced muscle mass, improved bone density, and increased metabolic rate. Drawing from both scientific research and practical experience, I provide tailored exercises that are safe, effective, and easily integrated into daily routines. I also address common concerns and misconceptions, offering strategies to overcome obstacles and ensure consistency. My goal is to inspire confidence and demonstrate that strength training is not only achievable but also transformative, enabling seniors to maintain their independence, enhance their mobility, and enjoy a higher quality of life. As a newbie to exercise or looking to refine your current regimen, this chapter serves as a comprehensive guide to building strength and fostering long-term health.

Building Upper Body Strength

Building upper body strength is essential for seniors to maintain independence, perform daily tasks with ease, and enhance overall quality of life. Strengthening the muscles in the arms, shoulders, and upper back not only supports better posture but also reduces the risk of falls and injuries. Engaging in regular upper body exercises can improve circulation, increase bone density, and contribute to a more robust immune system. Additionally, a strong upper body aids in activities such as lifting groceries, reaching for objects, and even simple movements like opening a door, making daily living more manageable and less strenuous.

One effective exercise for building upper body strength is Seated Arm Raises. This exercise targets the shoulder muscles, including the deltoids and trapezius, which are crucial for arm movement and stability. To perform Seated Arm Raises, sit comfortably in a sturdy chair with your feet flat on the floor. Slowly raise your arms out to the sides until they are parallel to the ground, holding the position for a few seconds before gently lowering them back down. This controlled movement helps in enhancing muscle tone and endurance without putting undue stress on the joints. Beginners can start with lighter weights or even no weights, gradually increasing resistance as strength improves.

Bicep Curls with Resistance Bands are another excellent exercise for seniors aiming to strengthen their upper arms. Bicep curls specifically target the biceps brachii, the muscles located at the front of the upper arm, which are essential for lifting and carrying objects. Using a resistance band provides a safe and adjustable way to add intensity to the exercise. To perform Bicep Curls, sit upright with your feet firmly planted. Hold the resistance band in both hands with your palms facing upward. Slowly curl your hands towards your shoulders, engaging the biceps, and then slowly extend your arms back to the starting position. This movement not only builds muscle strength but also enhances flexibility and coordination.

Shoulder Press Variations offer a versatile approach to strengthening the shoulders and upper back. This exercise engages the deltoids, triceps, and upper trapezius, contributing to improved arm strength and shoulder stability. To perform Shoulder Press Variations, sit comfortably with your back straight and feet flat on the floor. Hold a pair of light dumbbells or resistance bands at shoulder height with your palms facing forward. Slowly press the weights upward until your arms are fully extended, then lower them back to the starting position with control. Variations can include alternating arms or using different grips to target various muscle groups, ensuring a comprehensive workout for the upper body.

Incorporating these upper body exercises into a regular chair yoga routine can significantly enhance muscle strength, joint flexibility, and overall upper body functionality. It's important for seniors to start with manageable weights and resistance levels, gradually increasing intensity as their strength improves. Consistency is key; performing these exercises several times a week can lead to noticeable improvements in strength and endurance. Additionally, maintaining proper form and breathing techniques during each exercise ensures maximum effectiveness while minimizing the risk of injury. Consulting with a healthcare professional before beginning any new exercise regimen is advisable to ensure the exercises are appropriate for individual health conditions and fitness levels.

Building upper body strength through these chair-based exercises not only contributes to physical health but also fosters a sense of accomplishment and empowerment. As seniors develop greater strength and confidence in their abilities, they may find increased motivation to engage in other aspects of their fitness journey. Enhanced upper body strength can lead to better performance in daily activities, improved balance, and a higher quality of life. By dedicating time to these exercises, seniors can achieve significant health benefits, promoting longevity and sustained independence.

Enhancing Lower Body Strength

Enhancing lower body strength is crucial for seniors to maintain mobility, balance, and the ability to perform essential daily activities such as walking, climbing stairs, and standing up from a seated position. Strong lower body muscles, including the quadriceps, hamstrings, calves, and glutes, support joint health and reduce the risk of falls and fractures. Engaging in regular lower body exercises can also improve circulation, increase bone density, and boost overall physical stamina. Moreover, maintaining lower body strength contributes to better posture and a more active lifestyle, enhancing both physical and mental well-being.

Seated Leg Lifts are an effective exercise for strengthening the quadriceps and hip flexors, which are vital for leg movement and stability. To perform Seated Leg Lifts, sit upright in a sturdy chair with your feet flat on the floor. Slowly extend one leg out straight, holding the position for a few seconds before gently lowering it back down. Repeat the movement with the opposite leg. This exercise can be performed with or without ankle weights, depending on the individual's strength level. Seated Leg Lifts help in improving muscle tone, enhancing joint flexibility, and supporting overall lower body strength without placing excessive strain on the knees or hips.

Calf Raises and Extensions target the calf muscles, specifically the gastrocnemius and soleus, which play a key role in walking, standing, and maintaining balance. To perform Calf Raises, sit comfortably with your feet flat on the floor. Slowly lift your heels off the ground, rising onto the balls of your feet, and hold the position for a few seconds before lowering your heels back down. For Calf Extensions, extend one leg straight out in front of you, flexing your foot upward, and then return to the starting position. These exercises enhance ankle stability, improve circulation in the lower legs, and contribute to better overall leg strength, making everyday movements smoother and more controlled.

Thigh Squeezes and Extensions focus on the inner and outer thighs, as well as the hamstrings, which are essential for leg strength and stability. To perform Thigh Squeezes, place a small ball or pillow between your knees and gently squeeze your thighs together, holding the contraction for a few seconds before releasing. For Thigh Extensions, sit with your back straight and feet flat on the floor. Slowly extend one leg out straight, hold for a few seconds, and then return it to the starting position. These exercises help in toning the thigh muscles, enhancing joint stability, and supporting better overall lower body functionality, which is crucial for maintaining an active and independent lifestyle.

Incorporating these lower body exercises into a chair yoga routine provides seniors with a safe and effective way to build strength, improve mobility, and enhance overall lower body health. It is important to perform each exercise with proper form and controlled movements to maximize benefits and minimize the risk of injury. Seniors should start with a few repetitions and gradually increase the number as their strength improves. Consistency is essential; regular practice can lead to significant improvements in muscle tone, joint flexibility, and overall lower body strength. Additionally, combining these exercises with a balanced diet and adequate hydration can further support muscle health and overall well-being.

Enhancing lower body strength through these chair-based exercises not only improves physical capabilities but also contributes to better balance and coordination. Strong legs are fundamental for maintaining an upright posture, preventing falls, and supporting the body's weight during movement. As seniors develop greater lower body strength, they may experience increased confidence in their ability to navigate their environment independently and safely. This boost in physical strength can lead to greater participation in social activities, outdoor adventures, and other aspects of life that contribute to mental and emotional health. By dedicating time to these exercises, seniors can achieve lasting benefits that enhance their overall quality of life.

Core Strengthening Exercises

Core strengthening is a vital component of any fitness regimen, especially for seniors, as it supports balance, stability, and overall functional movement. A strong core encompasses the muscles in the abdomen, lower back, hips, and pelvis, which work together to maintain proper posture, support the spine, and facilitate everyday movements such as bending, twisting, and lifting. Strengthening these muscles can reduce the risk of falls, alleviate back pain, and improve overall mobility. Additionally, a robust core enhances athletic performance, aids in efficient breathing, and contributes to better coordination and balance, all of which are essential for maintaining independence and a high quality of life.

Seated Torso Twists are an effective exercise for engaging the oblique muscles and improving rotational flexibility in the spine. To perform Seated Torso Twists, sit upright in a sturdy chair with your feet flat on the floor and hands placed gently behind your head or crossed over your chest. Slowly rotate your upper body to the right, keeping your hips facing forward, and hold the position for a few seconds before returning to the center. Repeat the movement to the left side. This controlled twisting motion enhances spinal mobility, strengthens the abdominal muscles, and promotes better posture. Seated Torso Twists also help in reducing tension in the back and shoulders, contributing to overall spinal health and flexibility.

Abdominal Engagement Techniques focus on activating and strengthening the core muscles, including the rectus abdominis, transverse abdominis, and obliques. One such technique involves Seated Abdominal Contractions. To perform this exercise, sit comfortably with your back straight and feet flat on the floor. Place your hands on your abdomen and take a deep breath in, expanding your stomach. As you exhale, gently contract your abdominal muscles, pulling your belly button inward towards your spine. Hold the contraction for a few seconds before releasing and repeating the process. This exercise not only strengthens the abdominal muscles but also enhances breath control and promotes better core stability, which is essential for maintaining balance and preventing falls.

Gentle Seated Crunches provide a safe and effective way to strengthen the upper abdominal muscles without the strain associated with traditional crunches. To perform Gentle Seated Crunches, sit on the edge of a sturdy chair with your feet flat on the floor and your hands placed lightly behind your head or crossed over your chest. Slowly lean back, engaging your core muscles, and then return to the starting position by tightening your abdominal muscles. This controlled movement targets the upper abdominals, improves core strength, and enhances overall spinal support. Gentle Seated Crunches also promote better posture and can help alleviate lower back pain by strengthening the muscles that support the spine.

Incorporating these core strengthening exercises into a chair yoga routine provides seniors with a comprehensive approach to enhancing core stability, improving balance, and supporting overall physical health. It is important to perform each exercise with mindful attention to form and breathing, ensuring that the movements are controlled and deliberate. Seniors should start with a few repetitions and gradually increase the number as their core strength improves, always listening to their bodies and avoiding overexertion. Consistent practice of these exercises can lead to significant improvements in core strength, which in turn supports better posture, reduced back pain, and enhanced overall mobility. Additionally, a strong core contributes to better respiratory function and greater ease in performing daily activities, making these exercises an essential component of a well-rounded chair yoga routine.

Strengthening the core through these seated exercises not only enhances physical capabilities but also boosts confidence and independence. A strong core is fundamental for maintaining balance and stability, which are crucial for preventing falls and injuries. As seniors develop greater core strength, they may find it easier to engage in other physical activities, participate in social events, and enjoy a more active and fulfilling lifestyle. Moreover, the mental benefits of core strengthening, such as improved focus and reduced stress, contribute to overall well-being and a positive outlook on life. By dedicating time to these core exercises, seniors can achieve lasting benefits that support a healthy, active, and independent life.

Chapter 7

FLEXIBILITY AND MOBILITY

Maintaining flexibility and mobility is essential for seniors to ensure independence, reduce the risk of injuries, and enhance overall quality of life. This chapter delves into various techniques and practices within chair yoga that specifically target the improvement of range of motion and joint health. By incorporating these exercises into daily routines, seniors can experience significant enhancements in their physical capabilities and overall well-being.

Increasing Range of Motion

1. Seated Forward Bends

Seated forward bends are fundamental stretches in chair yoga that target the spine, hamstrings, and lower back. These movements help in elongating the muscles and improving flexibility, which is crucial for maintaining a healthy posture. For seniors, performing these bends while seated ensures stability and reduces the risk of falling, making the practice both safe and effective.

To begin, sit comfortably on the edge of the chair with your feet flat on the floor, hip-width apart. Inhale deeply, raising your arms overhead to lengthen your spine. As you exhale, slowly bend forward from the hips, reaching your hands toward your feet. It's important to keep the back straight and avoid hunching over, which ensures that the stretch is directed appropriately without causing strain.

Consistent practice of seated forward bends can lead to increased flexibility in the hamstrings and lower back, which in turn enhances overall mobility. This flexibility is particularly beneficial for daily activities such as bending down to tie shoes or picking up objects, reducing the likelihood of discomfort or injury. Additionally, forward bends can promote relaxation and alleviate stress, contributing to mental well-being.

For those with limited flexibility, modifications can be made to accommodate individual needs. Using a cushion or yoga strap can help in gradually increasing the depth of the stretch without overexertion. It's crucial to listen to the body and avoid pushing beyond comfortable limits, ensuring a safe and effective practice.

Incorporating seated forward bends into a daily routine can significantly improve range of motion over time. By prioritizing gentle and consistent stretching, seniors can maintain their physical independence and enjoy a higher quality of life. These exercises not only enhance flexibility but also promote a sense of accomplishment and confidence in one's physical abilities.

2. Side Stretches and Twists

Side stretches and twists are excellent for enhancing lateral flexibility and promoting spinal mobility. These exercises target the oblique muscles, shoulders, and lower back, contributing to a more balanced and flexible body. For seniors, performing these stretches in a seated position ensures safety while effectively improving range of motion.

To perform a seated side stretch, sit upright with your feet firmly planted on the ground. Inhale deeply and extend your right arm overhead, leaning gently to the left to feel a stretch along your right side. Hold this position for a few breaths, then switch sides, extending the left arm and leaning to the right. This movement helps in lengthening the sides of the torso and improving flexibility in the spine.

Seated twists add another dimension to flexibility by engaging the core muscles and enhancing spinal rotation. Begin by sitting tall with your feet flat on the floor. Inhale to prepare, and as you exhale, gently twist your upper body to the right, placing your left hand on the outside of your right thigh and your right hand on the back of the chair for support. Hold the twist for several breaths before returning to the center and repeating on the opposite side.

Regular practice of side stretches and twists can lead to improved posture and reduced stiffness in the back and shoulders. These exercises also aid in digestion and stimulate the internal organs, promoting overall health. Additionally, the rhythmic motion of twisting can have a calming effect on the mind, enhancing mental clarity and focus.

For those with limited mobility, modifications can be made to accommodate different levels of flexibility. Using a yoga strap or towel can assist in reaching the arms overhead, and performing smaller, controlled movements can help in gradually increasing the range of motion. It's essential to move slowly and mindfully, ensuring that each stretch is performed safely and effectively.

3. Gentle Spinal Rotations

Gentle spinal rotations are vital for maintaining the flexibility and health of the spine. These movements help in enhancing spinal mobility, reducing stiffness, and preventing discomfort associated with aging. For seniors, performing spinal rotations in a seated position ensures stability and minimizes the risk of injury while effectively targeting the back muscles.

To begin, sit comfortably with your feet flat on the floor and hands resting on your knees. Inhale deeply, lengthening your spine, and as you exhale, gently rotate your upper body to the right, keeping your hips facing forward. Hold the rotation for a few breaths, feeling the stretch along your spine and sides. Return to the center and repeat the movement to the left side, ensuring both sides are equally worked.

Spinal rotations improve the flexibility of the vertebrae and intervertebral discs, which is essential for maintaining a healthy spine. These exercises also engage the core muscles, providing additional support and stability to the back. Enhanced spinal mobility contributes to better posture and reduces the risk of back pain, which is common among seniors.

In addition to physical benefits, spinal rotations can have a positive impact on mental well-being. The rhythmic movement and focus required during the exercise promote mindfulness and relaxation, helping to alleviate stress and improve concentration. This dual benefit makes spinal rotations a valuable addition to a comprehensive chair yoga practice.

For those with limited spinal flexibility or experiencing discomfort, it's important to perform these rotations gently and within a comfortable range. Using a cushion or rolled towel behind the lower back can provide extra support and help in maintaining proper alignment. Always listen to your body and avoid forcing any movements, ensuring a safe and beneficial practice.

Incorporating gentle spinal rotations into daily routines can lead to significant improvements in spinal health and overall mobility. These exercises not only enhance physical flexibility but also contribute to a sense of mental clarity and relaxation, making them an essential component of chair yoga for seniors.

Joint Health and Mobility

1. Wrist and Ankle Circles

Maintaining joint health is crucial for seniors to ensure smooth and pain-free movements. Wrist and ankle circles are simple yet effective exercises that enhance the flexibility and strength of these joints. Performed in a seated position, these circles promote circulation and reduce stiffness, contributing to overall mobility and comfort.

To perform wrist circles, extend your arms forward with palms facing down. Slowly rotate your wrists in a circular motion, first clockwise and then counterclockwise. Start with small circles, gradually increasing the size as flexibility improves. This movement helps in loosening the wrist joints and increasing their range of motion, which is beneficial for daily activities like writing or eating.

Ankle circles follow a similar pattern. Lift one foot off the ground and rotate the ankle in a circular motion, first in one direction and then the other. Repeat the movement with the opposite foot. These circles enhance the flexibility of the ankle joints, which is essential for maintaining balance and stability during walking or standing.

Regular practice of wrist and ankle circles can prevent the onset of joint pain and stiffness, common issues faced by seniors. Improved joint mobility also contributes to better overall movement and reduces the risk of falls and injuries. Additionally, these exercises can alleviate discomfort caused by conditions like arthritis, making daily tasks more manageable.

For those experiencing significant joint pain or limited mobility, modifications can be made to accommodate their needs. Using a lightweight resistance band can add gentle resistance to the movements, enhancing strength without causing strain. It's important to perform these circles slowly and mindfully, ensuring that each motion is controlled and comfortable.

2. Hip Openers and Stretchers

Hip openers and stretchers are essential for maintaining the flexibility and mobility of the hip joints, which play a crucial role in overall movement and stability. These exercises target the muscles around the hips, including the glutes, hip flexors, and inner thighs, promoting better range of motion and reducing the risk of hip-related discomfort.

To begin, sit comfortably with your feet flat on the floor. Lift your right ankle and place it on your left knee, creating a figure-four shape. Gently press down on the right knee to deepen the stretch in the hip area. Hold this position for several breaths before switching to the opposite side. This figure-four stretch helps in opening the hips and relieving tension in the lower back.

Another effective hip opener is the seated butterfly stretch. Bring the soles of your feet together and let your knees fall outward, resembling the wings of a butterfly. Hold your ankles or feet and gently press your knees toward the floor, feeling a stretch in the inner thighs and hips. This movement enhances flexibility in the hip joints and improves circulation to the lower body.

Incorporating hip openers and stretchers into a regular chair yoga routine can lead to significant improvements in hip mobility and overall lower body flexibility. These exercises are particularly beneficial for seniors who spend a lot of time sitting, as they counteract the tightening of hip muscles that often occurs with prolonged inactivity.

For those with limited hip flexibility or experiencing pain, it's important to perform these stretches gently and within a comfortable range. Using a cushion or rolled towel under the knees can provide additional support and make the stretches more accessible. Always listen to your body and avoid forcing any movements, ensuring a safe and effective practice.

Regular hip openers and stretchers not only enhance joint mobility but also contribute to better posture and reduced lower back pain. By maintaining flexible and healthy hip joints, seniors can enjoy greater ease in daily activities such as walking, climbing stairs, and bending, thereby improving their overall quality of life.

3. Knee and Elbow Flexibility

Knee and elbow flexibility is pivotal for maintaining independence and performing everyday tasks with ease. Chair yoga offers targeted exercises that enhance the range of motion in these joints, promoting better functionality and reducing the risk of injuries. These movements are particularly beneficial for seniors, ensuring that the exercises are safe and accessible.

To improve knee flexibility, seated leg extensions are highly effective. Sit upright with both feet flat on the floor. Slowly extend your right leg straight out, keeping the heel on the ground and toes pointing upward. Hold the extended position for a few seconds before gently lowering the leg back down. Repeat the movement with the left leg. This exercise strengthens the quadriceps and enhances the flexibility of the knee joint, making movements like standing up and walking smoother.

Elbow flexibility can be improved through gentle arm bends and extensions. Begin by sitting comfortably with your arms relaxed by your sides. Slowly bend your right elbow, bringing your hand toward your shoulder, and then extend it back out straight. Repeat this movement several times before switching to the left arm. These exercises help in maintaining the range of motion in the elbow joints, which is essential for tasks such as lifting objects or performing daily chores.

Incorporating knee and elbow flexibility exercises into a regular chair yoga practice can lead to enhanced joint health and better overall mobility. These movements not only improve flexibility but also strengthen the surrounding muscles, providing additional support and stability to the joints. This dual benefit reduces the likelihood of joint pain and enhances the ability to perform daily activities with greater ease.

For seniors experiencing significant stiffness or discomfort, modifications can be made to accommodate their needs. Using a lightweight resistance band can add gentle resistance to the movements, enhancing strength without causing strain. It's important to perform these exercises slowly and mindfully, ensuring that each movement is controlled and comfortable.

Daily Mobility Practices

1. Integrating Yoga into Daily Routines

Integrating yoga into daily routines is essential for maintaining consistent flexibility and mobility gains. For seniors, incorporating chair yoga into everyday activities ensures that the benefits of yoga are sustained over time, promoting long-term health and well-being. By making yoga a regular part of the day, seniors can enjoy enhanced physical and mental health without significant disruptions to their schedules.

One effective way to integrate yoga into daily routines is by setting aside specific times for practice, such as morning stretches to start the day or evening relaxation sessions to unwind. These dedicated periods help in establishing a consistent habit, ensuring that yoga becomes a natural part of the daily routine. Additionally, short, frequent sessions can be more manageable and less intimidating for seniors, promoting adherence and enjoyment.

Another strategy is to incorporate yoga movements into existing activities. For example, performing gentle stretches while watching television or listening to music can make the practice more enjoyable and seamless. This approach ensures that yoga is not seen as an additional task but as a complementary activity that enhances daily living.

Creating a supportive environment is also crucial for integrating yoga into daily life. This can involve setting up a comfortable space with a sturdy chair and necessary accessories, such as cushions or yoga straps. A designated area encourages regular practice and makes it easier to maintain consistency, even amidst a busy schedule.

Ultimately, integrating yoga into daily routines empowers seniors to take control of their health and mobility. By making yoga a regular habit, seniors can experience sustained improvements in flexibility, strength, and overall well-being, leading to a more active and fulfilling lifestyle.

2. Simple Movements for Everyday Activities

Incorporating simple yoga movements into everyday activities can significantly enhance mobility and flexibility, making daily tasks easier and more enjoyable. These movements are designed to be subtle and unobtrusive, allowing seniors to reap the benefits of yoga without requiring dedicated time or space. By integrating these practices into routine activities, seniors can maintain their physical health and independence.

One example of a simple movement is seated leg lifts, which can be performed while sitting at a dining table or watching TV. Gently lifting and extending the legs helps in strengthening the lower body muscles and improving circulation. These subtle movements enhance mobility, making actions like standing up or walking more effortless and reducing the risk of falls.

Another effective movement is shoulder rolls, which can be done while engaged in conversations or reading. Slowly rolling the shoulders forward and backward helps in relieving tension and improving shoulder flexibility. This practice alleviates stiffness in the upper body, promoting better posture and reducing discomfort associated with prolonged sitting.

Incorporating deep breathing into daily activities is also beneficial. For instance, taking deep breaths while preparing meals or during short breaks can enhance lung capacity and promote relaxation. Deep breathing exercises improve oxygen flow to the muscles and brain, contributing to overall vitality and mental clarity.

By embedding these simple movements into daily life, seniors can maintain and even enhance their flexibility and mobility without the need for structured exercise sessions. These practices ensure that the benefits of yoga are continuously integrated into their lives, promoting sustained physical and mental well-being.

3. Maintaining Consistent Flexibility

Maintaining consistent flexibility is vital for seniors to ensure ongoing mobility and independence. Consistency in practicing chair yoga not only helps in preserving the gains achieved but also prevents the onset of stiffness and mobility issues. Establishing a regular routine and adopting strategies to stay motivated are key components of maintaining flexibility over the long term.

One effective way to maintain consistency is by setting realistic and achievable goals. Whether it's improving a specific stretch or increasing the duration of a yoga session, having clear objectives provides direction and motivation. Tracking progress through a journal or app can also help in recognizing improvements and staying committed to the practice.

Creating a supportive environment and community can further enhance consistency. Joining a chair yoga class or connecting with other seniors practicing yoga can provide encouragement and accountability. Sharing experiences and challenges with peers fosters a sense of camaraderie, making the practice more enjoyable and sustainable.

Incorporating variety into the yoga routine prevents monotony and keeps the practice engaging. Exploring different stretches, poses, and breathing techniques ensures that the body continues to adapt and improve. Variety also addresses different aspects of flexibility and mobility, promoting a more comprehensive approach to physical health.

Always learn to listen to your body and adapt to the practice as needed,this ensures that flexibility is maintained without causing strain or injury. Recognizing the signs of fatigue or discomfort and making necessary adjustments, such as taking breaks or modifying poses, promotes a safe and effective practice. By prioritizing consistency and mindfulness, seniors can enjoy sustained flexibility and mobility, enhancing their overall quality of life.

Chapter 8

POSTURE IMPROVEMENT

Good posture is fundamental to maintaining overall health and well-being, especially for seniors. Proper alignment of the body not only enhances physical appearance but also plays a crucial role in preventing discomfort and injuries. This chapter explores the importance of good posture, common postural issues faced by seniors, and the myriad benefits of improving posture through chair yoga. By understanding and applying these principles, seniors can achieve better alignment, reduce pain, and enhance their quality of life.

Understanding Good Posture

1. Importance of Proper Alignment

Proper alignment of the body is essential for maintaining balance and reducing the strain on muscles and joints. For seniors, maintaining correct posture can significantly impact their mobility and overall health. Proper alignment ensures that the body's weight is distributed evenly, minimizing the risk of developing musculoskeletal issues such as back pain, neck strain, and joint discomfort. Additionally, good posture supports the natural curves of the spine, promoting spinal health and flexibility.

Beyond physical benefits, proper alignment also influences mental well-being. When the body is aligned correctly, it can enhance breathing efficiency and circulation, leading to increased energy levels and reduced fatigue. This improved physical state can positively affect mood and cognitive function, contributing to a better quality of life. Furthermore, maintaining good posture can boost self-confidence and promote a sense of well-being, as individuals feel more poised and in control of their bodies.

In the context of chair yoga, understanding proper alignment is crucial for performing exercises safely and effectively. Each yoga pose is designed to align the body in a way that maximizes the benefits while minimizing the risk of injury. By focusing on alignment, seniors can ensure that they are getting the most out of their yoga practice, enhancing both physical and mental health. This mindful approach to alignment fosters a deeper connection between the mind and body, promoting overall harmony and balance.

Moreover, proper alignment can prevent the development of chronic conditions associated with poor posture. For example, slouching can lead to compressed organs and impaired digestion, while forward head posture can contribute to tension headaches and reduced lung capacity. By maintaining proper alignment, seniors can mitigate these risks and support their long-term health. This proactive approach to posture management is a key component of a holistic wellness strategy.

The importance of proper alignment extends beyond the immediate physical benefits. It lays the foundation for a healthier, more active lifestyle, enabling seniors to engage in daily activities with greater ease and comfort. By prioritizing alignment through chair yoga, seniors can enhance their mobility, reduce pain, and enjoy a more fulfilling and independent life.

2. Common Postural Issues in Seniors

As individuals age, various postural issues can arise due to natural changes in the body and lifestyle factors. Understanding these common postural problems is the first step toward addressing and correcting them. One prevalent issue is forward head posture, where the head juts forward relative to the shoulders. This misalignment can lead to neck strain, headaches, and decreased lung capacity, making breathing more difficult and reducing overall energy levels.

Another common postural issue among seniors is rounded shoulders, often resulting from prolonged periods of sitting or slouching. Rounded shoulders can cause tension in the upper back and neck, contributing to chronic pain and reduced range of motion. This posture can also impact the appearance of the chest, leading to a hunched or stooped look that affects self-esteem and confidence.

Additionally, seniors may experience a loss of spinal curvature, such as a decrease in the natural lumbar lordosis (inward curve of the lower back). This reduction can result in a flattened lower back, increasing the risk of lower back pain and stiffness. Changes in spinal curvature can also affect the alignment of other joints, leading to compensatory movements and further postural imbalances.

Pelvic tilt is another postural issue that can affect seniors. An anterior pelvic tilt, where the pelvis tilts forward, can cause the lower back to arch excessively, while a posterior pelvic tilt, where the pelvis tilts backward, can flatten the lower back. Both conditions can lead to discomfort, reduced mobility, and an increased risk of injury during daily activities. Addressing pelvic tilt through targeted exercises is essential for restoring balance and alignment.

Also, I want you to be aware that foot and ankle issues can also contribute to poor posture. Conditions such as plantar fasciitis or arthritis in the feet can alter the way a person stands and walks, leading to compensatory postural adjustments. These adjustments can create a chain reaction throughout the body, affecting the knees, hips, and spine. By recognizing and addressing these common postural issues, seniors can take proactive steps to improve their alignment and overall health through chair yoga.

3. Benefits of Improved Posture

Improving posture offers a wide range of benefits that significantly enhance the quality of life for seniors. One of the most immediate advantages is the reduction of pain and discomfort. Proper alignment alleviates pressure on the muscles and joints, decreasing the likelihood of chronic pain in areas such as the back, neck, and shoulders. This pain relief enables seniors to engage more comfortably in daily activities and enjoy a more active lifestyle.

Enhanced respiratory function is another key benefit of improved posture. When the body is aligned correctly, the chest and diaphragm have more room to expand, allowing for deeper and more efficient breathing. This increased lung capacity can lead to better oxygenation of the blood, boosting energy levels and overall vitality. Improved breathing also contributes to reduced stress and anxiety, promoting a sense of calm and well-being.

Better digestion is also linked to improved posture. When the spine is properly aligned, the internal organs are not compressed, allowing the digestive system to function more effectively. This can alleviate issues such as acid reflux, constipation, and bloating, leading to improved digestive health. A healthy digestive system plays a crucial role in overall wellness, supporting nutrient absorption and immune function.

In addition to physical benefits, improved posture positively impacts mental health. Good posture is associated with increased self-esteem and confidence, as individuals feel more poised and in control of their bodies. This positive self-image can enhance social interactions and contribute to a more optimistic outlook on life. Furthermore, the focus and mindfulness required to maintain proper posture can enhance cognitive function and mental clarity, supporting overall mental well-being.

Improved posture supports long-term health and independence. By maintaining proper alignment, seniors can preserve their mobility and reduce the risk of falls and injuries. This preservation of mobility is essential for maintaining independence and the ability to perform daily tasks without assistance. Overall, the benefits of improved posture extend beyond immediate physical comfort, contributing to a healthier, more active, and fulfilling life for seniors.

Seated Posture Correction

1. Aligning Your Spine

Aligning the spine is fundamental to achieving good posture and overall spinal health. In a seated position, proper spinal alignment ensures that the natural curves of the spine are maintained, reducing the risk of discomfort and injury. For seniors, who may spend extended periods sitting, whether for meals, reading, or engaging in chair yoga, maintaining spinal alignment is crucial for preventing chronic pain and enhancing mobility.

To begin aligning the spine, sit comfortably at the edge of the chair with both feet flat on the floor. Distribute your weight evenly across both hips and ensure that your knees are at a 90-degree angle, aligned with your hips. Sit back in the chair, allowing the backrest to support the natural curve of your lower back. This position helps in maintaining the lumbar lordosis, preventing the lower back from slumping forward.

Engaging the core muscles is another essential aspect of spinal alignment. Gently tighten the abdominal muscles without holding your breath, creating a supportive base for the spine. This engagement helps in stabilizing the upper body and reducing the strain on the lower back. Maintaining a slight engagement of the core throughout seated activities promotes continuous spinal support and alignment.

Head and neck alignment also play a vital role in spinal alignment. Keep your head level, ensuring that your ears are aligned with your shoulders. Avoid tilting your head forward or backward, as this can create unnecessary tension in the neck and upper back. By maintaining a neutral head position, you support the entire spine, promoting a balanced and aligned posture.

Regular awareness and adjustment are key to maintaining spinal alignment. Periodically check your posture throughout the day, making minor adjustments as needed to stay aligned. Incorporating mindful practices, such as chair yoga, can help in developing a habit of maintaining proper alignment effortlessly. Over time, these adjustments become second nature, contributing to sustained spinal health and overall well-being.

2. Adjusting Chair Height and Position

The height and position of the chair are critical factors in achieving and maintaining good posture. An improperly adjusted chair can lead to misalignment of the spine, discomfort, and increased strain on muscles and joints. For seniors, who may have specific needs regarding support and accessibility, ensuring that the chair is correctly adjusted is paramount for a safe and effective yoga practice.

To start, adjust the chair height so that your feet are flat on the floor with your knees bent at a 90-degree angle. This position helps in aligning the hips and knees, promoting a balanced posture. If the chair is too high, use a footrest to ensure that your feet are adequately supported. Conversely, if the chair is too low, consider adding cushions to raise your seating position without compromising comfort.

The depth of the chair seat is another important consideration. When seated, there should be a small gap between the back of your knees and the edge of the seat. This spacing allows for proper circulation and prevents pressure on the back of the knees, enhancing comfort and reducing the risk of numbness or swelling. If necessary, use additional padding or adjust the chair's position to achieve the optimal seat depth.

Back support is crucial for maintaining spinal alignment. Choose a chair with a supportive backrest that follows the natural curve of your spine. If the chair lacks adequate support, consider using a lumbar cushion or rolled towel placed at the lower back to maintain the natural lumbar curve. Proper back support helps in preventing slouching and encourages a straight and aligned posture during yoga exercises.

The chair's stability and mobility should be considered. Ensure that the chair is sturdy and does not wobble, providing a secure base for yoga movements. If the chair has wheels, consider locking them in place to prevent unintended movement during exercises. A stable and well-positioned chair enhances safety and allows seniors to perform yoga poses with confidence and ease, maximizing the benefits of their practice.

3. Engaging Core Muscles for Support

Engaging the core muscles is essential for providing support to the spine and maintaining good posture during seated activities. The core comprises the abdominal muscles, lower back, and pelvis, which work together to stabilize the body and facilitate movement. For seniors, strengthening the core through chair yoga can enhance balance, reduce the risk of falls, and improve overall mobility.

To engage the core, begin by sitting upright in the chair with your feet flat on the floor and knees bent at a 90-degree angle. Take a deep breath in, expanding your abdomen, and as you exhale, gently draw your navel toward your spine without holding your breath. This action activates the deep abdominal muscles, providing a stable foundation for the upper body. Maintaining this gentle engagement throughout seated activities helps in supporting the spine and reducing strain on the lower back.

Incorporating core engagement into yoga poses can further strengthen these muscles. For example, during a seated twist, engaging the core helps in maintaining balance and control, allowing for a deeper and more effective stretch. Similarly, during seated leg lifts, a strong core provides the necessary support to lift the legs without causing undue stress on the lower back. This integration of core strength into various exercises enhances overall stability and posture.

Breathing exercises also play a role in engaging the core. Deep, diaphragmatic breathing naturally activates the core muscles, promoting relaxation and reducing tension. Practicing mindful breathing while maintaining core engagement helps in creating a harmonious connection between the mind and body, enhancing the benefits of both the breathing and yoga practices. This mindful approach supports sustained core strength and improved posture.

Regularly incorporating core engagement into daily routines, such as sitting and standing movements, can lead to significant improvements in core strength and spinal support. As seniors become more adept at engaging their core muscles, they will experience enhanced balance, reduced back pain, and increased confidence in their movements. A strong core is a cornerstone of good posture, contributing to long-term health and independence.

It's important to approach core engagement with patience and consistency. Strengthening the core muscles takes time and regular practice, especially for seniors who may have experienced muscle loss or weakness. Chair yoga provides a safe and accessible way to gradually build core strength, allowing seniors to progress at their own pace and achieve lasting benefits. By prioritizing core engagement, seniors can enjoy improved posture, enhanced stability, and a greater sense of well-being.

Exercises for Better Posture

1. Seated Cat-Cow Stretch

The Seated Cat-Cow Stretch is a fundamental yoga exercise that enhances spinal flexibility and promotes good posture. This gentle movement helps in mobilizing the spine, relieving tension in the back and neck, and encouraging mindful breathing. For seniors, performing this stretch in a seated position ensures stability and safety while reaping the benefits of spinal flexibility and relaxation.

To perform the Seated Cat-Cow Stretch, begin by sitting comfortably at the edge of the chair with your feet flat on the floor and hands resting on your knees. Inhale deeply, arching your back and lifting your chest and head toward the ceiling (Cow Pose). This movement opens the chest and stretches the front of the body, promoting an upright and open posture. Hold the pose for a few breaths, feeling the expansion of the spine and the elongation of the torso.

As you exhale, round your spine, tucking your chin toward your chest and drawing your belly in (Cat Pose). This motion flexes the spine, releasing tension in the back and neck, and gently massages the abdominal organs. The Cat Pose helps in neutralizing the spine and preparing it for the next inhale, creating a fluid and rhythmic movement that synchronizes with the breath.

Repeat the Seated Cat-Cow Stretch several times, moving slowly and mindfully with each breath. Focus on the sensations in your spine and the flow of your breath, allowing yourself to fully experience the benefits of each movement. This mindful approach enhances the connection between the mind and body, promoting relaxation and mental clarity alongside physical flexibility.

Incorporating the Seated Cat-Cow Stretch into your daily chair yoga routine can lead to improved spinal mobility, reduced back pain, and enhanced posture. This simple yet effective exercise serves as a foundation for more advanced yoga poses, building the strength and flexibility necessary for maintaining good posture. By regularly practicing this stretch, seniors can enjoy a healthier spine and a more balanced, aligned posture.

2. Chest Openers and Shoulder Blends

Chest openers and shoulder blends are essential exercises for counteracting the effects of slouching and rounded shoulders, common postural issues among seniors. These movements help in stretching and strengthening the muscles of the chest and shoulders, promoting a more open and upright posture. By incorporating these exercises into chair yoga, seniors can alleviate tension, improve upper body flexibility, and enhance overall posture.

To perform a seated chest opener, start by sitting tall in the chair with your feet flat on the floor. Clasp your hands behind your back, interlacing your fingers or holding onto the chair back for support. Inhale deeply, squeezing your shoulder blades together and lifting your chest toward the ceiling. This movement stretches the chest and shoulders, counteracting the tendency to hunch forward. Hold the pose for several breaths, feeling the openness in your upper body.

Shoulder blends complement the chest openers by targeting the shoulder muscles and promoting flexibility in the upper back. To perform shoulder blends, sit comfortably with your feet flat and arms relaxed by your sides. Inhale, lifting your shoulders toward your ears, and as you exhale, roll them back and down in a circular motion. Repeat this movement several times, coordinating it with your breath to release tension and improve shoulder mobility.

Another effective exercise is the Seated Arm Stretch. Extend your right arm straight out in front of you at shoulder height, palm facing down. Use your left hand to gently press against the right arm, guiding it across your body toward the left side. Hold the stretch for a few breaths, feeling the stretch in your right shoulder and upper back. Repeat on the opposite side, ensuring both sides are equally worked.

Regular practice of chest openers and shoulder blends can lead to significant improvements in upper body flexibility and posture. These exercises help in reducing tightness in the chest and shoulders, making it easier to maintain an upright and aligned posture throughout the day. Additionally, these movements enhance circulation to the upper body, promoting overall health and reducing the risk of musculoskeletal issues.

Incorporating these exercises into a daily chair yoga routine ensures that seniors can effectively address and correct postural imbalances. By consistently practicing chest openers and shoulder blends, individuals can achieve a more open and relaxed upper body, enhancing both their physical comfort and overall posture. These exercises are simple, accessible, and highly beneficial, making them an essential component of a comprehensive posture improvement strategy.

3. Neck and Upper Back Strengtheners

Strengthening the neck and upper back is crucial for maintaining good posture and preventing discomfort in these areas. Weakness in these muscles can lead to slouching, tension headaches, and chronic pain, which are common issues among seniors. Chair yoga offers targeted exercises that enhance the strength and flexibility of the neck and upper back, promoting an upright and aligned posture.

One effective exercise is the Seated Neck Stretch. Begin by sitting comfortably with your feet flat on the floor and shoulders relaxed. Gently tilt your head to the right, bringing your ear toward your shoulder without raising the shoulder. To deepen the stretch, you can place your right hand on the left side of your head and apply gentle pressure. Hold the stretch for a few breaths, feeling the release in the left side of your neck. Repeat on the opposite side to ensure balanced flexibility.

Another beneficial exercise is the Upper Back Squeeze. Sit upright with your feet firmly planted and hands resting on your thighs. Inhale deeply, reaching your arms forward with palms facing each other. As you exhale, squeeze your shoulder blades together, pulling your arms back while keeping them straight. This movement engages the upper back muscles, strengthening them and promoting better posture. Hold the squeeze for a few seconds before releasing and repeating the exercise.

The Seated Row is an excellent exercise for building upper back strength. To perform a seated row, sit tall in the chair with your feet flat and knees bent. Extend your arms forward, palms facing down. Inhale and pull your elbows back, drawing your hands toward your torso while squeezing your shoulder blades together. Exhale as you slowly extend your arms back to the starting position. This exercise targets the rhomboids and latissimus dorsi, essential muscles for maintaining an upright posture.

Incorporating these neck and upper back strengtheners into your chair yoga routine can lead to improved muscle tone and reduced tension in the upper body. Strengthened neck and upper back muscles support the spine, reducing the risk of postural imbalances and associated pain. Additionally, these exercises enhance overall upper body flexibility, making it easier to maintain proper alignment throughout daily activities.

Regular practice of neck and upper back strengthening exercises not only improves posture but also contributes to overall spinal health. By building strength in these areas, seniors can experience greater ease in movements, reduced discomfort, and enhanced physical confidence. These exercises are simple to perform, require minimal equipment, and offer significant benefits, making them a valuable addition to any chair yoga practice focused on posture improvement.

Chapter 9

JOINT HEALTH AND PAIN RELIEF

I understand that maintaining joint health and managing pain are crucial for sustaining an active and fulfilling life, especially for those of us over 70. This chapter delves into the transformative power of chair yoga in addressing common joint issues such as arthritis, chronic pain, and reduced mobility. Drawing from both personal experiences and extensive research, I provide practical strategies and gentle exercises designed to alleviate discomfort, enhance flexibility, and strengthen the muscles surrounding the joints. This chapter offers a comprehensive approach to reducing inflammation, improving range of motion, and preventing further joint deterioration, all tailored to the unique needs of seniors. My goal is to empower you with the knowledge and tools necessary to achieve greater comfort and mobility, enabling you to enjoy everyday activities with ease and confidence. If you're dealing with persistent pain or looking to prevent future joint issues, it serves as your essential resource for achieving optimal joint health through the accessible and supportive practice of chair yoga.

Managing Arthritis with Yoga

Gentle Movements for Joint Comfort

Arthritis is a common condition that causes inflammation and stiffness in the joints, which can be particularly challenging for seniors. Chair yoga offers gentle movements that help improve joint comfort without overstraining the body. Simple exercises like seated cat-cow stretches or side stretches can increase flexibility and range of motion in the shoulders, hips, and knees. These gentle movements promote circulation, which can reduce the stiffness often felt in arthritic joints. When practiced regularly, these movements help ease discomfort and encourage the joints to move more freely.

Reducing Inflammation Through Stretching

Arthritis is often accompanied by inflammation, which can exacerbate pain and restrict movement. Chair yoga incorporates various stretches that target areas prone to inflammation, such as the knees, elbows, and wrists. Stretching encourages blood flow, which helps to reduce swelling and improve joint function. For instance, gentle leg stretches or wrist rotations can help decrease tension and soothe inflammation in the affected areas. By incorporating anti-inflammatory stretches into the routine, individuals can experience a noticeable reduction in swelling and improved comfort.

Strengthening Surrounding Muscles

Building strength around the affected joints is a key component of arthritis management, and yoga can play an important role in this. Chair yoga focuses on strengthening the muscles that support the joints, such as the quadriceps for the knees, the core for the back, and the upper arms for the shoulders. Stronger muscles help take pressure off the joints, making movements easier and less painful. Chair poses like seated leg lifts or arm raises can be performed with controlled breathing to strengthen muscles without straining them. Strengthening the muscles around arthritic joints provides greater stability and reduces the risk of injury.

Improving Posture and Alignment

Good posture is essential for joint health, especially for individuals with arthritis. Poor posture can lead to additional strain on the joints, particularly in the spine and hips. Chair yoga helps seniors improve posture by promoting proper alignment of the body. Exercises such as seated spinal twists and shoulder rolls help to lengthen the spine, open the chest, and relieve pressure from the lower back. As posture improves, the load on the joints is more evenly distributed, reducing pain and preventing further damage to the joints. Better posture also encourages a greater sense of balance and stability in daily activities.

Breathwork for Pain Relief

Breathing techniques are an integral part of yoga and can help manage arthritis-related pain. Deep, mindful breathing helps relax the nervous system, which can reduce the perception of pain. In chair yoga, incorporating breathing exercises like diaphragmatic breathing or alternate nostril breathing can help soothe the mind and alleviate the tension held in the body. By pairing breathwork with movement, seniors can reduce muscle tightness and stress, which can be especially helpful in managing arthritis pain. Controlled breathing enhances the effects of each pose and allows for deeper relaxation, providing pain relief in a natural way.

Alleviating Chronic Pain

Techniques for Back and Neck Pain

Chronic pain in the back and neck is common as individuals age, often caused by muscle imbalances or poor posture. Chair yoga offers specific techniques to relieve discomfort in these areas by targeting the muscles and joints that support the spine. Gentle stretches like seated forward bends or neck rolls can help release tightness and improve flexibility. These exercises focus on lengthening the spine, which helps to alleviate pressure on the lower back and neck. Regular practice can help reduce muscle stiffness, improve alignment, and minimize discomfort in the back and neck.

Managing Knee and Hip Discomfort

Knee and hip pain can be particularly debilitating for seniors, often caused by conditions like arthritis or overuse. Chair yoga includes low-impact movements designed to relieve pain and improve mobility in these areas. Seated leg extensions, knee lifts, and gentle hip stretches help to strengthen the muscles around the knees and hips, providing better support and reducing discomfort. These movements also help maintain joint lubrication, which is essential for healthy joints. By incorporating these exercises into their routine, seniors can experience improved mobility and a reduction in pain over time.

Shoulder and Elbow Pain Relief

Shoulder and elbow pain are common complaints for seniors, often resulting from repetitive movements or poor posture. Chair yoga can be highly effective in alleviating pain in these areas through gentle stretching and strengthening exercises. Shoulder rolls, arm lifts, and elbow bends help increase circulation, reduce stiffness, and improve flexibility in the shoulders and elbows. These exercises can also help alleviate tension in the upper back and neck, which can contribute to shoulder discomfort. By strengthening the muscles around the shoulders and elbows, seniors can enjoy greater range of motion and reduced pain in their daily activities.

Releasing Muscle Tension

Chronic pain is often accompanied by tight muscles, which can worsen the discomfort over time. Chair yoga focuses on releasing muscle tension through mindful stretching and relaxation techniques. Regularly practicing seated stretches for the legs, back, and arms can help release built-up tension in the muscles and fascia. For example, seated twists and gentle side stretches help to elongate the spine and relax the muscles around the torso. By incorporating these stretches into their routine, seniors can experience significant relief from muscle tightness, which in turn helps to alleviate chronic pain.

Mind-Body Connection for Pain Management

Yoga is not just about physical movement; it also emphasizes the mind-body connection. Chronic pain is often exacerbated by stress and anxiety, which can increase muscle tension and heighten the perception of pain. Chair yoga encourages seniors to be present in the moment, focusing on their breath and sensations in the body. This mindfulness practice can help reduce pain by calming the nervous system and improving emotional well-being. By learning to manage the mind-body connection through yoga, seniors can develop coping mechanisms for dealing with chronic pain, leading to an overall sense of relaxation and relief.

Enhancing Joint Mobility

Range of Motion Exercises

Maintaining and improving joint mobility is essential for seniors to remain independent and active. Chair yoga includes a variety of exercises designed to enhance the range of motion in the joints, especially those that are prone to stiffness, such as the hips, knees, and shoulders. For example, seated leg circles and shoulder shrugs help to increase the flexibility and movement in these key areas. These exercises allow the joints to move through their full range of motion, helping to prevent stiffness and improve overall mobility. By practicing these movements regularly, seniors can enjoy greater freedom in their everyday activities.

Lubricating Joints with Movement

Joints require lubrication to move smoothly and without discomfort. Regular movement is one of the most effective ways to keep joints lubricated, and chair yoga offers low-impact exercises that do just that. Simple movements like seated marches, knee bends, and wrist rotations promote the production of synovial fluid, which helps reduce friction and keep the joints healthy. These exercises are particularly beneficial for seniors with osteoarthritis or other joint conditions, as they help maintain joint health and reduce the risk of further damage. Lubricating the joints through movement can also improve mobility and reduce pain in the long run.

Preventative Practices for Joint Health

Preventing joint problems before they arise is crucial for maintaining long-term joint health. Chair yoga encourages preventative practices that help seniors protect their joints and maintain flexibility. For example, proper alignment during seated poses helps to prevent excessive wear and tear on the joints. Additionally, strengthening exercises for the muscles surrounding the joints, such as leg lifts and seated squats, help support the joints and reduce the risk of injury. By focusing on joint health in a preventative way, seniors can maintain their mobility and avoid painful conditions like arthritis or bursitis.

Improving Flexibility for Joint Function

Flexibility plays a key role in maintaining joint function, and chair yoga helps enhance flexibility in a safe and controlled manner. Regular stretching exercises help lengthen the muscles and increase flexibility around the joints, which in turn improves overall joint function. Exercises like seated hamstring stretches or ankle rolls target areas that are prone to tightness and stiffness, promoting better movement in the hips, knees, and ankles. Flexibility is essential not only for improving mobility but also for preventing falls and injuries, which can be a major concern for seniors. Chair yoga provides a gentle yet effective way to keep the body flexible and the joints functioning properly.

Building Balance and Stability

Joint mobility is closely tied to balance and stability, which are crucial for seniors' overall health and safety. Chair yoga includes exercises that help improve balance by focusing on strengthening the core and lower body muscles. For example, seated leg lifts and heel-to-toe walking strengthen the muscles that support the joints and improve coordination. By practicing these balance-enhancing exercises, seniors can reduce their risk of falls, which is a common cause of joint injuries in older adults. Improving balance also allows seniors to move with greater confidence and control, further enhancing their joint health and mobility.

These exercises and techniques are designed to support joint health and pain relief in seniors over 70, offering a safe and effective way to manage discomfort, improve mobility, and maintain an active lifestyle.

Chapter 10

WEIGHT MANAGEMENT AND YOGA

I am passionate about demonstrating how yoga can be a transformative tool for weight management, especially for seniors seeking a gentle yet effective approach to maintaining a healthy weight. In this chapter, I delve into the unique ways yoga supports weight loss and overall wellness by combining mindful movement, breathing techniques, and mental focus. I explore tailored yoga routines that accommodate varying fitness levels and physical capabilities, ensuring that each exercise not only burns calories but also enhances flexibility, strength, and balance. Additionally, I discuss the importance of integrating yoga with healthy eating habits and lifestyle choices to create a sustainable weight management plan. Through personal anecdotes, scientific insights, and practical tips, I aim to empower you to embrace yoga as a holistic practice that nurtures both body and mind, ultimately leading to a healthier, more vibrant life. Whether you are new to yoga or looking to deepen your practice, this chapter provides the guidance and inspiration needed to achieve your weight management goals with grace and confidence.

Yoga for Weight Loss

Calorie-Burning Seated Exercises

Weight management is a significant aspect of maintaining overall health, especially for seniors. Chair yoga offers a variety of seated exercises that effectively burn calories without the need for strenuous movements or standing poses. These exercises are designed to engage multiple muscle groups simultaneously, promoting increased heart rate and energy expenditure. For example, seated marches, where you lift your knees alternately while sitting, can elevate your heart rate and burn calories effectively. Additionally, arm movements such as seated punches or overhead reaches engage the upper body, further contributing to calorie burning.

Incorporating resistance elements, such as using light weights or resistance bands, can enhance the calorie-burning potential of seated exercises. For instance, performing seated bicep curls or shoulder presses not only strengthens muscles but also increases metabolic rate. These activities, when performed consistently, can lead to significant improvements in weight management over time. It's important to start with manageable repetitions and gradually increase intensity to avoid strain or injury.

Another effective calorie-burning exercise is the seated twist, which engages the core muscles and promotes flexibility. By twisting the torso from side to side while keeping the hips stationary, seniors can work their abdominal muscles and improve spinal mobility. This movement not only aids in calorie burning but also enhances overall body coordination and balance. Additionally, integrating breathing techniques with these exercises can further amplify their effectiveness by increasing oxygen intake and promoting relaxation.

Consistency is key when it comes to burning calories through chair yoga. Establishing a regular routine that includes a mix of cardiovascular and strength-building exercises ensures that all major muscle groups are engaged. This balanced approach not only aids in weight loss but also contributes to improved muscle tone and joint health. Moreover, performing these exercises in a controlled and mindful manner helps prevent overexertion and reduces the risk of injury, making chair yoga a safe and sustainable option for weight management.

Calorie-burning seated exercises provide a practical and accessible way for seniors to manage their weight. By integrating these movements into daily routines, individuals can achieve their weight loss goals while enjoying the numerous health benefits that yoga offers. From enhancing metabolism to improving flexibility and strength, chair yoga serves as a comprehensive tool for maintaining a healthy weight and promoting overall well-being.

Enhancing Metabolism Through Movement

Metabolism plays a crucial role in weight management, as it determines how efficiently the body converts food into energy. As we age, metabolic rates naturally decline, making it more challenging to maintain or lose weight. Chair yoga can help counteract this decline by incorporating movements that stimulate metabolic processes. Engaging in regular chair yoga sessions increases muscle mass, which in turn boosts metabolic rate since muscle tissue burns more calories at rest compared to fat tissue.

In addition to building muscle, certain chair yoga poses and sequences are specifically designed to activate the body's metabolic pathways. Dynamic movements, such as seated sun salutations or flowing sequences that combine stretching and strengthening, can elevate heart rate and enhance metabolic activity. These exercises encourage the body to utilize stored energy, thereby aiding in weight loss and preventing weight gain.

Breathing techniques, an integral part of yoga, also contribute to metabolic enhancement. Practices like pranayama, which involve controlled and mindful breathing, improve oxygen intake and circulation. Efficient oxygenation of the body's tissues supports better cellular function and energy production. This heightened metabolic activity not only aids in burning calories but also promotes overall vitality and energy levels, which are essential for an active lifestyle.

Nutrition plays a complementary role in enhancing metabolism through yoga. Consuming a balanced diet rich in lean proteins, whole grains, and fresh vegetables provides the necessary nutrients to support metabolic functions. Pairing these dietary habits with regular chair yoga practice creates a synergistic effect, optimizing the body's ability to burn calories and maintain a healthy weight. Seniors should focus on nutrient-dense foods that provide sustained energy without excessive calories, supporting both weight management and overall health.

Consistency and progression are vital for maintaining an elevated metabolic rate through chair yoga. Gradually increasing the intensity and variety of exercises ensures that the body continues to adapt and respond positively. Incorporating new poses, extending the duration of sessions, or adding resistance can help sustain metabolic improvements over time. By making chair yoga a regular part of their routine, seniors can effectively enhance their metabolism, supporting long-term weight management and improved health outcomes.

Combining Yoga with Nutrition

Effective weight management is not solely dependent on physical activity; nutrition plays an equally important role. Combining chair yoga with a balanced diet creates a holistic approach to weight loss, addressing both the physical and dietary aspects of health. Seniors should focus on consuming a variety of nutrient-rich foods that provide the necessary vitamins, minerals, and macronutrients to support their yoga practice and overall well-being.

A well-rounded diet for weight management includes ample lean proteins, which are essential for muscle repair and growth. Incorporating sources such as chicken, fish, legumes, and tofu can help maintain muscle mass, especially when paired with strength-building chair yoga exercises. Additionally, whole grains like brown rice, quinoa, and whole wheat bread provide sustained energy for yoga sessions, preventing fatigue and enhancing performance.

Fruits and vegetables should form the cornerstone of a senior's diet, offering a plethora of vitamins, antioxidants, and fiber. These nutrients support metabolic functions, reduce inflammation, and promote satiety, making it easier to manage calorie intake. Including a variety of colorful produce ensures that seniors receive a broad spectrum of nutrients, which can enhance their overall health and complement the physical benefits of chair yoga.

Healthy fats are also crucial for a balanced diet, contributing to brain health and hormone production. Sources such as avocados, nuts, seeds, and olive oil should be included in meals to provide essential fatty acids that support cellular function and energy levels. These fats help in the absorption of fat-soluble vitamins, further enhancing the nutritional benefits of a balanced diet. Combining these dietary elements with regular yoga practice maximizes the effectiveness of weight management efforts.

Hydration is another key component of combining yoga with nutrition. Adequate water intake ensures that the body functions optimally, aiding in digestion, nutrient absorption, and the elimination of toxins. Seniors should aim to drink sufficient water throughout the day, especially before and after yoga sessions, to stay hydrated and maintain energy levels. By integrating mindful eating practices with regular chair yoga, seniors can achieve sustainable weight loss and enjoy improved health and vitality.

Building a Sustainable Routine

Setting Realistic Weight Goals

Setting realistic weight goals is essential for maintaining motivation and achieving long-term success in weight management. Seniors should begin by assessing their current weight and understanding their body's unique needs. Consulting with healthcare professionals can provide valuable insights into what constitutes a healthy weight range, taking into account factors such as age, height, and overall health status. Realistic goals are those that are achievable and sustainable, rather than drastic changes that may lead to frustration or health issues.

When setting weight goals, it's important to focus on gradual progress rather than immediate results. Aiming for a modest weight loss of 1-2 pounds per week is generally considered safe and attainable. This approach allows the body to adjust to changes without causing undue stress or requiring extreme dietary restrictions. Additionally, setting incremental milestones can help seniors celebrate small victories, maintaining their motivation and commitment to their weight management journey.

Incorporating non-scale victories into goal setting can also enhance motivation. These victories include improvements in flexibility, strength, energy levels, and overall well-being, all of which are achievable through regular chair yoga practice. By recognizing and valuing these achievements, seniors can maintain a positive outlook and stay committed to their weight management goals, even when the scale may not reflect immediate changes.

Personalizing weight goals ensures that they align with individual lifestyles and preferences. Seniors should consider their daily routines, physical capabilities, and personal interests when setting their goals. For instance, integrating chair yoga sessions that they enjoy and can realistically commit to will increase the likelihood of adherence. Flexibility in goal setting allows for adjustments as needed, accommodating changes in health status or lifestyle without derailing progress.

Maintaining a positive and patient mindset is crucial when setting weight goals. Understanding that weight management is a gradual process helps seniors stay resilient in the face of challenges. Emphasizing consistency, perseverance, and self-compassion over perfection encourages a healthier relationship with weight loss. By setting realistic, personalized goals, seniors can build a sustainable routine that supports their weight management efforts and enhances their overall quality of life.

Tracking Progress and Staying Motivated

Tracking progress is a fundamental aspect of maintaining motivation and ensuring continued success in weight management. Seniors can utilize various methods to monitor their progress, such as keeping a journal, using mobile apps, or maintaining a visual chart. Recording daily yoga sessions, dietary intake, and physical changes provides a comprehensive view of their journey, highlighting both achievements and areas needing improvement. This practice not only reinforces accountability but also offers valuable insights into patterns and progress over time.

In addition to tracking weight and measurements, documenting non-scale indicators of progress can be highly motivating. These indicators include increased flexibility, improved strength, enhanced mood, and better sleep quality. By acknowledging these positive changes, seniors can appreciate the broader benefits of their yoga practice, fostering a sense of accomplishment that extends beyond numerical weight loss. Celebrating these milestones encourages continued dedication and a positive mindset.

Staying motivated requires setting short-term and long-term goals that provide direction and purpose. Short-term goals, such as completing a certain number of yoga sessions each week or mastering a new pose, offer immediate targets to strive for. Long-term goals, like achieving a specific weight or maintaining a consistent yoga routine for several months, provide a broader vision for sustained effort. Balancing these goals helps maintain enthusiasm and prevents burnout, ensuring that seniors remain engaged in their weight management journey.

Creating a supportive environment plays a crucial role in maintaining motivation. Engaging with friends, family members, or fellow yoga practitioners can provide encouragement and accountability. Sharing progress, challenges, and successes with a supportive community fosters a sense of belonging and mutual motivation. Additionally, seeking guidance from a yoga instructor or joining a chair yoga class can offer structured support, enhancing commitment and enjoyment.

Incorporating variety and creativity into the routine helps prevent monotony and keeps the practice enjoyable. Exploring different chair yoga routines, trying new poses, or integrating music and meditation can make each session unique and engaging. By keeping the yoga practice fresh and interesting, seniors are more likely to stay motivated and committed to their weight management goals. Embracing change and adapting the routine as needed ensures that the journey remains fulfilling and effective over the long term.

Adapting Exercises for Ongoing Success

As seniors progress in their weight management journey, it is essential to adapt and modify exercises to continue challenging the body and preventing plateaus. Adapting chair yoga exercises involves adjusting the intensity, duration, and complexity of movements to match the evolving fitness levels and goals. For example, increasing the number of repetitions, holding poses for longer periods, or incorporating resistance elements like light weights can enhance the effectiveness of the exercises. These modifications ensure that the body continues to respond positively, promoting ongoing weight loss and fitness improvements.

Listening to the body is crucial when adapting exercises to prevent overexertion and injury. Seniors should pay close attention to how their bodies feel during and after yoga sessions, making adjustments as needed. If a particular pose causes discomfort or strain, modifying it to a more comfortable version or reducing the intensity can help maintain safety and sustainability. This mindful approach allows for gradual progression, ensuring that the yoga practice remains beneficial without causing harm.

Incorporating new chair yoga poses and routines keeps the practice dynamic and engaging. Exploring different styles of chair yoga, such as incorporating elements of tai chi or gentle stretching, can add variety and interest. Learning new poses challenges the body in different ways, promoting comprehensive fitness and preventing boredom. Additionally, seeking inspiration from various sources, such as yoga videos, books, or classes, can provide fresh ideas and techniques to integrate into the routine.

Setting new goals and revisiting existing ones is another way to adapt exercises for ongoing success. As seniors achieve their initial weight management goals, establishing new targets keeps the journey forward-moving and purposeful. These new goals might include enhancing flexibility, building greater strength, or achieving a higher level of cardiovascular fitness. By continuously setting and pursuing new objectives, seniors maintain a sense of progress and achievement, fueling their motivation to persist in their yoga practice.

Seeking professional guidance when adapting exercises can provide personalized support and expertise. Working with a certified chair yoga instructor ensures that modifications are appropriate and effective, tailored to individual needs and capabilities. Instructors can offer valuable feedback, suggest new techniques, and help troubleshoot any challenges that arise. This professional support enhances the adaptability and effectiveness of the yoga practice, ensuring that seniors continue to thrive in their weight management journey and enjoy the full benefits of chair yoga.

Balancing Diet and Yoga

Nutritional Tips for Seniors

Maintaining a balanced diet is a cornerstone of effective weight management, particularly when combined with a regular chair yoga practice. Seniors should focus on consuming nutrient-dense foods that provide essential vitamins, minerals, and macronutrients to support their overall health and fitness goals. Incorporating a variety of fruits, vegetables, lean proteins, whole grains, and healthy fats ensures that the body receives the necessary nutrients for energy, muscle maintenance, and metabolic function.

One key nutritional tip for seniors is to prioritize protein intake, which is vital for muscle repair and growth. Including sources such as poultry, fish, beans, lentils, and dairy products can help maintain muscle mass, especially when engaging in strength-building chair yoga exercises. Additionally, plant-based proteins offer a healthy alternative that can support weight management while providing essential amino acids. Balancing protein intake throughout the day aids in sustained energy levels and prevents muscle loss associated with aging.

Fiber-rich foods play a significant role in weight management by promoting satiety and supporting digestive health. Whole grains, legumes, fruits, and vegetables are excellent sources of dietary fiber, helping seniors feel fuller for longer periods and reducing the likelihood of overeating. Incorporating these foods into meals can aid in controlling calorie intake while providing necessary nutrients for overall health. Additionally, fiber supports regular bowel movements and reduces the risk of digestive issues, contributing to a healthier and more comfortable lifestyle.

Hydration is another critical aspect of a balanced diet for seniors. Adequate water intake ensures that the body functions optimally, supporting digestion, nutrient absorption, and toxin elimination. Seniors should aim to drink at least eight glasses of water a day, adjusting as needed based on activity levels and individual health conditions. Incorporating hydrating foods, such as cucumbers, watermelon, and citrus fruits, can also contribute to overall fluid intake, enhancing hydration without excessive calorie consumption.

Seniors should be mindful of portion sizes and mindful eating practices to maintain a balanced diet. Understanding appropriate portion sizes helps prevent overeating and supports weight management efforts. Eating slowly and paying attention to hunger and fullness cues can enhance the enjoyment of meals and prevent unnecessary calorie intake. By implementing these nutritional tips, seniors can create a sustainable and balanced diet that complements their chair yoga practice, promoting effective weight management and overall well-being.

Hydration and Its Importance

Hydration is a fundamental aspect of maintaining good health, particularly for seniors engaged in regular physical activity like chair yoga. Adequate hydration supports numerous bodily functions, including temperature regulation, joint lubrication, and nutrient transportation. Water is essential for digestion, absorption of nutrients, and the elimination of waste products, making it a critical component of overall health and effective weight management.

Dehydration can lead to a range of health issues that can hinder weight management efforts. Symptoms such as fatigue, dizziness, and muscle cramps can impair the ability to perform chair yoga exercises effectively. Moreover, dehydration can slow down metabolism and reduce the body's ability to burn calories efficiently. Ensuring adequate fluid intake helps maintain energy levels, supports physical performance, and enhances the effectiveness of yoga sessions, contributing to successful weight management.

Seniors should aim to drink water consistently throughout the day, rather than waiting until they feel thirsty, which is a sign that dehydration may already be occurring. Carrying a water bottle during yoga sessions and taking regular sips can help maintain hydration levels. Additionally, incorporating herbal teas, infused water, and water-rich foods like cucumbers, strawberries, and oranges can contribute to overall fluid intake without adding excessive calories or sugars.

It is important to recognize that certain factors, such as medications, medical conditions, and environmental conditions, can affect hydration needs. Seniors should consult with healthcare professionals to determine their specific hydration requirements and make adjustments as necessary. For instance, individuals with kidney issues or those taking diuretics may need to increase their fluid intake to compensate for increased water loss. Personalized hydration plans ensure that each senior meets their unique needs, supporting both their yoga practice and weight management goals.

Understanding the signs of dehydration and responding promptly is crucial for maintaining optimal health. Symptoms such as dry mouth, dark urine, and reduced skin elasticity indicate the need for increased fluid intake. By staying attuned to their bodies and prioritizing hydration, seniors can enhance their overall well-being, support their weight management efforts, and maximize the benefits of their chair yoga practice. Consistent and mindful hydration practices ensure that the body remains well-nourished and capable of performing daily activities with ease and comfort.

Mindful Eating Practices

Mindful eating is a powerful tool for weight management, particularly when combined with a regular chair yoga practice. This approach involves paying full attention to the experience of eating, including the taste, texture, and aroma of food, as well as recognizing hunger and fullness cues. For seniors, mindful eating can help develop a healthier relationship with food, prevent overeating, and enhance overall satisfaction with meals.

One key aspect of mindful eating is slowing down the pace of meals. Taking the time to chew thoroughly and savor each bite allows the body to register fullness signals more effectively, reducing the likelihood of overeating. Seniors can practice mindful eating by setting aside dedicated time for meals, minimizing distractions such as television or smartphones, and focusing entirely on the act of eating. This deliberate approach fosters a deeper appreciation for food and promotes better digestion and nutrient absorption.

Another important element of mindful eating is being aware of emotional triggers that may lead to unhealthy eating habits. Stress, boredom, or loneliness can sometimes drive individuals to eat for reasons other than hunger. By practicing mindfulness, seniors can become more attuned to their emotional states and develop healthier coping mechanisms that do not involve food. Techniques such as deep breathing, meditation, or gentle chair yoga stretches can be integrated into mealtime routines to address emotional needs without resorting to overeating.

Portion control is also a crucial component of mindful eating. Seniors can benefit from using smaller plates, measuring serving sizes, and being conscious of the amount of food they consume. This awareness helps prevent excessive calorie intake and supports weight management efforts. Additionally, incorporating a variety of colorful and nutrient-dense foods ensures that meals are both satisfying and nourishing, reducing the temptation to reach for unhealthy snacks or oversized portions.

Reflecting on the eating experience can enhance mindful eating practices. Taking a few moments after each meal to assess how the body feels, whether it's satisfied, energized, or still hungry, helps reinforce mindful eating habits. This reflection encourages seniors to make informed choices about their food intake, aligning their eating patterns with their weight management and overall health goals. By embracing mindful eating, seniors can enjoy their meals more fully, support their chair yoga practice, and achieve sustainable weight management with greater ease and satisfaction.

Chapter 11

BALANCE AND STABILITY

My goal in this part is to empower you, our esteemed senior readers, with the confidence and physical foundation necessary to navigate daily life with grace and assurance. Throughout my years of practicing and teaching chair yoga, I've witnessed firsthand how enhancing balance and stability can significantly reduce the risk of falls, improve posture, and foster a sense of independence. In this chapter, I will guide you through a series of carefully designed exercises that strengthen your core, improve coordination, and increase your overall stability—all from the comfort and safety of your chair. By incorporating these practices into your routine, you will not only enhance your physical balance but also boost your mental resilience, allowing you to move through each day with greater ease and confidence. Together, we will explore the transformative power of balance-focused chair yoga, ensuring that you maintain a strong, stable foundation for years to come.

Improving Seated Balance

Stabilizing Techniques

Maintaining balance while seated is fundamental for seniors to ensure safety and enhance overall mobility. Stabilizing techniques begin with proper alignment, ensuring that the spine is straight and the feet are firmly planted on the ground. Adjusting the chair to the correct height allows for optimal support, reducing the risk of slumping or leaning, which can lead to instability. Incorporating subtle movements, such as shifting weight from side to side or gently rocking forward and backward, helps to engage the muscles that support balance. Additionally, using armrests can provide extra support during exercises, offering a secure point to hold onto and preventing falls.

Core Engagement for Better Balance

A strong core is essential for maintaining balance, both while seated and during movement. Engaging the core muscles involves activating the abdominal and lower back muscles to provide stability and support to the spine. Simple exercises like seated torso twists or gentle abdominal contractions can significantly enhance core strength over time. Consistent core engagement not only improves balance but also contributes to better posture and reduced back pain. Encouraging seniors to focus on their breathing while engaging the core can further enhance the effectiveness of these exercises, promoting a mind-body connection that is crucial for balance.

Seated Balance Challenges

Introducing balance challenges in a seated position can help seniors gradually build their stability and confidence. These challenges can include exercises such as lifting one foot off the ground while keeping the other firmly planted or extending the arms forward and holding the position for a few seconds. Another effective challenge is to slowly open and close the legs while maintaining an upright posture, which engages multiple muscle groups simultaneously. These exercises should be performed slowly and mindfully, allowing individuals to gauge their comfort levels and progress at their own pace. Over time, these challenges can lead to noticeable improvements in balance and coordination.

Incorporating Dynamic Movements

Dynamic movements within seated yoga routines add variety and further enhance balance by engaging different muscle groups. Movements such as seated marching, where one lifts the knees alternately, or arm circles, which involve rotating the arms in circular motions, can improve both balance and cardiovascular health. These dynamic exercises encourage continuous muscle activation, which is vital for maintaining balance and preventing stiffness. Additionally, incorporating dynamic movements can make the exercise sessions more engaging and enjoyable, motivating seniors to stay consistent with their practice.

Monitoring Progress and Adjusting Techniques

Tracking progress is essential to ensure that the balance and stability exercises are effective and to make necessary adjustments. Seniors can keep a simple journal noting their daily or weekly performance, such as the number of repetitions or the duration of each exercise. Observing improvements in balance, such as reduced swaying or increased confidence while performing tasks, can provide positive reinforcement. If certain exercises become too easy, modifications can be made to increase their difficulty, such as adding resistance with lightweight bands or increasing the duration of holds. Regularly assessing and adjusting techniques ensures that the exercises remain challenging and beneficial.

Transitioning to Standing (When Ready)

Safe Stand-Up Techniques

Transitioning from a seated to a standing position requires careful attention to ensure safety and prevent falls. Seniors should start by positioning their feet flat on the floor, shoulder-width apart, to provide a stable base. Before standing, it's important to engage the core and slowly lean forward, using the arms to push off the chair's arms if available. Gradual movements, avoiding sudden jerks or rapid shifts, help maintain balance during the transition. Practicing this technique regularly can build the necessary strength and confidence to stand independently, reducing reliance on support and enhancing overall mobility.

Assisted Balance Exercises

Assisted balance exercises are invaluable for seniors who are not yet ready to stand unaided. These exercises involve using props such as a sturdy table, countertop, or even a partner for support. For instance, practicing partial stand-ups by leaning forward with the support of a table can help develop the muscles needed for full standing. Another effective exercise is to hold onto a stable surface while performing gentle leg lifts, which strengthens the lower body and improves balance. Assisted exercises provide the necessary support while still challenging the muscles, facilitating a safe progression towards standing independently.

Gradual Progression to Standing Poses

Gradual progression is key to successfully transitioning to standing poses without compromising safety. Starting with small movements, such as shifting weight from one foot to the other while seated, can prepare the body for more significant shifts involved in standing. As strength and balance improve, seniors can begin incorporating simple standing poses like the Mountain Pose or the Tree Pose, using support as needed. Introducing these poses gradually allows the body to adapt to new movements and builds the confidence required to perform them independently. Consistent practice ensures steady progress, making standing poses a natural and comfortable part of the yoga routine.

Strengthening Lower Body Muscles

Strong lower body muscles are crucial for maintaining balance and stability during standing and movement. Exercises focused on the legs, such as seated leg lifts, calf raises, and gentle squats using the chair for support, can significantly enhance muscle strength. Strengthening these muscles not only aids in standing but also improves the ability to perform daily activities with greater ease. Incorporating resistance bands or light weights can add an extra challenge, further promoting muscle growth and endurance. A robust lower body provides a solid foundation for balance, reducing the risk of falls and enhancing overall mobility.

Building Confidence and Reducing Fear

Fear of falling can be a significant barrier to improving balance and mobility in seniors. Building confidence through consistent practice and positive reinforcement is essential. Starting with simple exercises and gradually increasing their complexity allows seniors to experience small successes, boosting their self-assurance. Encouraging a supportive environment, whether through group classes or the presence of a caregiver, can also alleviate anxiety related to movement. Positive affirmations and celebrating progress, no matter how minor, contribute to a positive mindset, making the transition to standing poses a more enjoyable and less intimidating experience.

Preventing Falls and Injuries

Awareness and Proprioception

Awareness of one's body position and movements, known as proprioception, plays a critical role in preventing falls and injuries. Proprioception involves the brain's ability to perceive the position and movement of the body in space, which is essential for maintaining balance. Chair yoga enhances proprioception through mindful movements and focused breathing, helping seniors become more attuned to their body's signals. Exercises that involve slow, deliberate motions encourage greater body awareness, enabling individuals to react more effectively to shifts in balance. Improved proprioception not only aids in preventing falls but also enhances coordination and movement efficiency.

Strengthening Support Muscles

Strengthening the muscles that support balance is a proactive strategy for fall prevention. Targeting specific muscle groups, such as the quadriceps, hamstrings, and calf muscles, can provide the necessary support for maintaining an upright posture and executing movements safely. Seated exercises like leg extensions, knee lifts, and ankle circles effectively engage these muscles without the need for standing. Additionally, upper body strength exercises, such as arm raises and shoulder presses, contribute to overall stability. Consistent strengthening of support muscles enhances the body's resilience against slips and trips, reducing the likelihood of falls and related injuries.

Creating a Safe Exercise Environment

A safe exercise environment is paramount to preventing falls and injuries during chair yoga practice. Ensuring that the area around the chair is free from obstacles, such as loose rugs, clutter, or sharp objects, minimizes the risk of tripping. Adequate lighting is essential to prevent missteps, especially in the evening or in low-light settings. Using a chair with sturdy arms provides additional support and stability during exercises, offering a reliable point of contact in case of imbalance. Additionally, placing a non-slip mat under the chair can prevent sliding, ensuring that the chair remains stationary throughout the practice. Creating a secure and comfortable environment allows seniors to focus on their exercises without undue worry about potential hazards.

Incorporating Fall Prevention Strategies

Integrating specific fall prevention strategies into the chair yoga routine can significantly enhance safety. This includes teaching seniors how to fall safely by practicing controlled movements and understanding how to use their hands to break a fall if necessary. Educating about the importance of wearing appropriate footwear and removing unnecessary obstacles from the home environment further contributes to fall prevention. Additionally, encouraging regular vision and hearing check-ups ensures that sensory impairments do not compromise balance and awareness. By incorporating these strategies, chair yoga becomes not only a tool for improving balance but also a comprehensive approach to reducing the risk of falls and promoting long-term safety.

Chapter 12

MINDFULNESS AND MENTAL CLARITY

I have witnessed firsthand the profound impact that mindfulness can have on enhancing mental clarity and overall well-being, especially for seniors. In this chapter, I explore in details the transformative practices of mindfulness within the context of chair yoga, offering techniques that not only calm the mind but also sharpen focus and promote emotional balance. Drawing from both scientific research and personal experiences, I guide you through simple yet powerful exercises that integrate deep breathing, meditation, and present-moment awareness. These practices are designed to help you navigate the challenges of aging with grace and resilience, reducing stress and anxiety while fostering a sense of inner peace and cognitive sharpness. You are new to mindfulness or looking to deepen your existing practice, this chapter provides the tools and insights needed to achieve greater mental clarity and a more centered, fulfilling life.

Mind-Body Connection in Yoga

Enhancing Awareness Through Movement

The mind-body connection is a fundamental aspect of yoga, emphasizing the seamless integration of mental and physical well-being. In chair yoga, this connection becomes even more significant, as the limited movement encourages a deeper focus on internal sensations and mental states. By engaging in deliberate movements, seniors can cultivate a heightened sense of body awareness, enabling them to recognize and respond to their bodies' needs more effectively. This enhanced awareness not only improves physical health but also fosters a greater sense of self-understanding and mindfulness.

Movement in chair yoga serves as a medium through which individuals can explore their physical limits and capabilities without the strain associated with standing or lying down exercises. Each stretch and pose is performed with intentionality, encouraging practitioners to pay close attention to how their bodies feel in different positions. This mindfulness during movement helps in identifying areas of tension, stiffness, or discomfort, allowing for adjustments that promote better alignment and comfort. Over time, this practice can lead to improved posture, reduced pain, and increased flexibility.

Moreover, enhancing awareness through movement has profound psychological benefits. As seniors become more attuned to their bodies, they also develop a greater awareness of their emotional states. The slow, deliberate motions of chair yoga provide a calming rhythm that can soothe the mind, reducing anxiety and promoting emotional balance. This dual focus on the body and mind creates a harmonious state of well-being, where physical health and mental clarity support each other synergistically.

In addition to personal awareness, mindful movement in chair yoga can improve cognitive functions such as concentration and memory. Engaging in yoga requires focusing on specific actions, breathing patterns, and bodily sensations, which exercises the brain and enhances neural connectivity. This mental engagement helps in maintaining cognitive sharpness, making chair yoga an excellent practice for seniors aiming to preserve their mental faculties as they age.

The practice of enhancing awareness through movement fosters a sense of empowerment and independence. By understanding their bodies better, seniors can take proactive steps in managing their health and well-being. This self-awareness encourages a more active role in their fitness routines, leading to sustained engagement and long-term benefits. Ultimately, chair yoga becomes not just a physical exercise but a comprehensive practice that nurtures the mind, body, and spirit.

Techniques for Mental Focus

Maintaining mental focus is essential for achieving the full benefits of chair yoga, especially for seniors who may experience age-related cognitive decline. Techniques for enhancing mental focus in yoga involve strategies that sharpen attention, reduce distractions, and promote a state of mental clarity. These techniques are designed to be gentle yet effective, making them accessible and beneficial for seniors engaging in chair yoga.

One effective technique for improving mental focus is the practice of mindful breathing. By concentrating on the breath, individuals can anchor their attention in the present moment, minimizing wandering thoughts and enhancing concentration. Deep, rhythmic breathing exercises help in calming the mind, creating a stable foundation for focused movement. This practice not only aids in maintaining mental clarity during yoga sessions but also extends its benefits into daily life, fostering a more centered and attentive mindset.

Another valuable technique is the use of guided intentions. Setting specific intentions before beginning a yoga session provides a clear mental goal, directing focus towards meaningful objectives. Whether the intention is to cultivate gratitude, seek relaxation, or enhance physical strength, having a purpose helps in maintaining concentration throughout the practice. This deliberate focus enriches the yoga experience, making each session more purposeful and engaging.

Visualization is also a powerful tool for enhancing mental focus. By imagining serene landscapes, peaceful environments, or positive outcomes, seniors can create a mental sanctuary that supports concentration and relaxation. Visualization techniques guide the mind away from distractions, fostering a deeper connection between the body and mind. This practice not only enhances focus during yoga but also contributes to overall mental well-being by promoting positive thinking patterns.

Additionally, incorporating mindful listening into chair yoga can significantly improve mental focus. Paying close attention to the sounds within and around oneself—such as the breath, the subtle movements of the body, or ambient noises—encourages a heightened state of awareness. This attentive listening cultivates a deeper presence, enabling seniors to stay engaged and focused throughout their yoga practice. Over time, mindful listening can enhance cognitive functions and promote a more attentive and alert mind.

The practice of regular meditation complements chair yoga by further enhancing mental focus. Even brief periods of meditation can train the mind to maintain attention and resist distractions. By integrating meditation with yoga, seniors can develop a robust mental discipline that supports sustained concentration and mental clarity. This combination not only enriches the yoga practice but also provides tools for managing daily challenges with a focused and calm mindset.

Benefits of Mindfulness Practices

Mindfulness practices within chair yoga offer a multitude of benefits that extend beyond physical health, significantly enhancing mental and emotional well-being. For seniors, incorporating mindfulness into their yoga routine can lead to improved cognitive functions, reduced stress levels, and a greater sense of overall happiness. These benefits are particularly valuable as individuals age, providing a holistic approach to maintaining a high quality of life.

One of the primary benefits of mindfulness in chair yoga is the reduction of stress and anxiety. By focusing on the present moment and engaging in mindful movements, seniors can experience a sense of calm and relaxation. This mental state helps in lowering cortisol levels, the hormone associated with stress, thereby promoting a more peaceful and balanced emotional state. Regular mindfulness practice can lead to long-term improvements in managing stress, contributing to better mental health and resilience.

Moreover, mindfulness enhances emotional regulation, allowing seniors to navigate their feelings with greater ease and stability. Through mindful awareness, individuals become more attuned to their emotional states, recognizing and addressing negative emotions before they escalate. This heightened emotional intelligence fosters a more positive outlook on life, reducing feelings of loneliness, depression, and anxiety that are common in older age. As a result, mindfulness practices can significantly improve emotional well-being and contribute to a happier, more fulfilling life.

In addition to emotional benefits, mindfulness practices in chair yoga can enhance cognitive functions such as memory, attention, and problem-solving skills. Engaging in mindful activities stimulates the brain, promoting neuroplasticity—the brain's ability to form new neural connections. This cognitive stimulation is crucial for seniors, as it helps in maintaining mental sharpness and delaying age-related cognitive decline. By regularly practicing mindfulness, seniors can keep their minds active and agile, supporting overall brain health.

Physical benefits are also closely tied to mindfulness in yoga. Mindful movements promote better body awareness, leading to improved posture, balance, and coordination. This heightened awareness helps in preventing falls and injuries, a significant concern for seniors. Additionally, mindfulness encourages a more intentional approach to movement, reducing the risk of overexertion and promoting sustainable exercise habits. These physical benefits contribute to enhanced mobility, independence, and overall quality of life.

I want you to know that mindfulness practices foster a deeper connection between the mind and body, promoting a sense of unity and harmony. This integrative approach to health encourages seniors to view their bodies as dynamic and responsive, capable of achieving wellness through mindful engagement. By nurturing this connection, mindfulness empowers individuals to take an active role in their health and well-being, leading to a more balanced and enriched life. In essence, the benefits of mindfulness in chair yoga encompass every aspect of an individual's life, making it an invaluable practice for seniors seeking comprehensive well-being.

Stress Reduction Through Yoga

Relaxation Techniques

Relaxation is a cornerstone of effective stress management, and chair yoga offers a variety of techniques tailored to the needs of seniors. These relaxation methods are designed to soothe the nervous system, reduce muscle tension, and promote a sense of calm and tranquility. By integrating these techniques into their daily routine, seniors can effectively manage stress and enhance their overall well-being.

One fundamental relaxation technique in chair yoga is the Progressive Muscle Relaxation (PMR). This method involves systematically tensing and then relaxing different muscle groups, starting from the feet and moving upwards to the head. By focusing on the contrast between tension and relaxation, seniors can become more aware of areas in their bodies that hold stress. This awareness allows them to consciously release tension, promoting physical relaxation and mental calmness.

Another effective technique is the Guided Relaxation practice, where individuals are led through a series of calming visualizations and soothing instructions. This method helps seniors detach from daily stressors and immerse themselves in a peaceful mental space. Guided relaxation can be particularly beneficial for those who find it challenging to relax on their own, providing structure and direction to their relaxation efforts. Over time, this practice can enhance the ability to enter a state of relaxation more easily and frequently.

Mindful Breathing is also a key relaxation technique in chair yoga. By focusing on the breath, seniors can anchor their attention in the present moment, reducing the impact of stress-inducing thoughts. Techniques such as deep diaphragmatic breathing or the 4-7-8 breathing method help in slowing the heart rate and lowering blood pressure, promoting a state of physiological relaxation. Consistent practice of mindful breathing can lead to long-term improvements in stress resilience and emotional regulation.

Additionally, the use of Aromatherapy during relaxation sessions can amplify the calming effects of chair yoga. Incorporating soothing scents like lavender, chamomile, or eucalyptus can enhance the sensory experience, further promoting relaxation. Aromatherapy stimulates the olfactory system, which is closely linked to the limbic system—the part of the brain responsible for emotions and memory. This sensory enhancement can deepen the relaxation response, making the practice more effective and enjoyable for seniors.

Gentle Stretching and Movement integrated with relaxation can enhance the overall stress-reducing benefits of chair yoga. Slow, deliberate movements help in releasing physical tension while maintaining a state of mental calmness. Combining stretching with relaxation techniques ensures that the body remains comfortable and supported, preventing strain and promoting a holistic sense of well-being. This integrative approach ensures that both the mind and body benefit from the relaxation practices, leading to a comprehensive reduction in stress levels.

Breathing for Calmness

Breathing is a powerful tool in managing stress, and chair yoga places a strong emphasis on breathing techniques to foster calmness and relaxation. Proper breathing not only enhances physical health by improving oxygen flow and circulation but also plays a crucial role in regulating the nervous system and promoting mental tranquility. For seniors, mastering breathing techniques can be particularly beneficial in mitigating the effects of stress and enhancing overall quality of life.

One of the most effective breathing techniques for calmness is Diaphragmatic Breathing, also known as belly breathing. This technique involves deep inhalations that expand the diaphragm, allowing the lungs to fully fill with air. Seniors can practice diaphragmatic breathing by placing one hand on the chest and the other on the abdomen, ensuring that the abdomen rises more than the chest during inhalation. This method encourages full oxygen exchange, which slows the heartbeat and stabilizes blood pressure, inducing a state of relaxation.

Alternate Nostril Breathing is another technique that promotes balance and calmness. This method involves breathing in through one nostril while closing the other, then switching sides with each breath. Alternate nostril breathing helps in harmonizing the left and right hemispheres of the brain, fostering a balanced and peaceful mental state. For seniors, this technique can enhance focus and reduce mental clutter, making it easier to maintain calmness throughout the day.

Box Breathing, also known as square breathing, is a structured technique that can significantly reduce stress and promote mental clarity. This method involves inhaling for a count of four, holding the breath for four, exhaling for four, and holding again for four. The rhythmic nature of box breathing helps in regulating the breath and calming the mind, making it an excellent practice for seniors looking to manage stress effectively. Consistent practice of box breathing can lead to improved emotional regulation and a greater sense of inner peace.

Incorporating Pursed-Lip Breathing can also aid in achieving calmness. This technique involves inhaling slowly through the nose and exhaling through tightly pressed lips, as if blowing out a candle. Pursed-lip breathing helps in controlling the breath, making exhalation longer than inhalation, which promotes relaxation and reduces anxiety. For seniors, especially those with respiratory concerns, this method can enhance breathing efficiency while simultaneously fostering a sense of calm.

Mindful Breathing Meditation integrates breathing techniques with meditation to deepen the state of calmness. During this practice, seniors focus solely on their breath, observing each inhalation and exhalation without judgment or distraction. This heightened focus on the breath helps in quieting the mind, reducing the impact of stressors, and promoting a profound sense of relaxation. Mindful breathing meditation not only aids in immediate stress reduction but also builds long-term resilience against future stressors, contributing to sustained mental well-being.

Guided Visualization Exercises

Guided visualization is a powerful technique within chair yoga that leverages the mind's ability to create vivid mental images to promote relaxation and mental clarity. This practice involves imagining serene and positive scenarios, which can help in reducing stress, enhancing mood, and fostering a sense of inner peace. For seniors, guided visualization exercises offer a safe and effective way to escape daily stressors and cultivate a more positive mental state.

One common guided visualization exercise involves imagining a peaceful natural setting, such as a quiet beach, a lush forest, or a tranquil garden. By visualizing the sights, sounds, and sensations of these environments, seniors can transport their minds away from stressful thoughts and into a place of calm and serenity. This mental escape not only provides immediate relaxation but also creates a mental sanctuary that individuals can return to whenever they need a respite from stress.

Another effective visualization technique focuses on the concept of Healing Light. In this exercise, seniors imagine a warm, glowing light surrounding their body, penetrating deep into their muscles and joints to alleviate pain and tension. This visualization promotes a sense of healing and rejuvenation, complementing the physical benefits of chair yoga. By visualizing the healing light, individuals can enhance their body's natural ability to recover and maintain health, fostering both physical and mental well-being.

Goal-Oriented Visualization is a technique that combines visualization with intention-setting. Seniors can visualize themselves achieving specific goals, such as improving flexibility, maintaining balance, or managing chronic pain. By creating a clear mental image of their desired outcomes, individuals can strengthen their motivation and commitment to their yoga practice. This positive reinforcement not only enhances the effectiveness of the exercises but also boosts self-confidence and a sense of accomplishment.

Additionally, Affirmation-Based Visualization integrates positive affirmations with mental imagery. Seniors can repeat affirming statements, such as "I am strong and flexible" or "I am calm and centered," while visualizing themselves embodying these qualities. This combination reinforces positive self-beliefs and encourages a more optimistic outlook on life. Affirmation-based visualization helps in reshaping negative thought patterns, promoting mental clarity and emotional resilience.

Guided Visualization for Emotional Release focuses on letting go of negative emotions and fostering emotional healing. Seniors can visualize releasing stress, anger, or sadness by imagining these emotions being carried away by a gentle breeze or dissolving into the air. This practice provides a safe and controlled way to process and release pent-up emotions, contributing to improved mental health and emotional balance. Guided visualization for emotional release not only alleviates stress but also promotes a sense of liberation and inner harmony.

Enhancing Cognitive Function

Yoga Practices for Brain Health

Maintaining cognitive function is crucial for seniors, and chair yoga offers several practices specifically designed to support brain health. These practices engage both the body and mind, promoting neural connectivity, enhancing cognitive flexibility, and protecting against age-related cognitive decline. By integrating these yoga practices into their routine, seniors can sustain mental acuity and overall brain vitality.

One key yoga practice for brain health is Coordination and Synchronization of Breath with Movement. This practice involves performing seated yoga poses in harmony with the breath, creating a rhythmic flow that stimulates brain activity. Coordinating breath and movement enhances neural communication and stimulates the brain's executive functions, such as planning, decision-making, and problem-solving. This synchronization not only improves physical coordination but also keeps the brain engaged and active.

Memory-Boosting Poses are another essential component of chair yoga for cognitive enhancement. Poses that require concentration and recall, such as repeating sequences of movements or holding poses for specific durations, challenge the brain and improve memory retention. By regularly practicing these poses, seniors can strengthen their memory pathways, making it easier to remember information and perform daily tasks with greater efficiency.

Mindful Movement Exercises also play a significant role in supporting brain health. These exercises emphasize slow, deliberate movements that require focus and attention, encouraging the brain to remain active and engaged. Mindful movement promotes neuroplasticity, the brain's ability to form new neural connections, which is vital for learning and adapting to new information. This continual stimulation helps in maintaining cognitive flexibility and reducing the risk of cognitive decline.

Furthermore, Balance and Coordination Exercises within chair yoga contribute to brain health by stimulating the cerebellum, the part of the brain responsible for coordination and balance. Engaging in exercises that challenge balance, even while seated, activates neural pathways that support motor skills and spatial awareness. Improved balance and coordination not only enhance physical stability but also support cognitive functions related to movement and spatial orientation.

Meditative Practices Integrated with Yoga provide a dual benefit for brain health. Meditation enhances focus, reduces stress, and promotes mental clarity, while yoga engages the body in cognitive activities. This combination creates a synergistic effect that boosts overall brain function. Regular meditation and yoga practices have been shown to increase gray matter density in the brain, which is associated with improved memory, emotional regulation, and cognitive resilience. By incorporating these practices, seniors can significantly enhance their cognitive health and maintain mental sharpness.

Memory and Concentration Enhancements

Memory and concentration are critical cognitive functions that can decline with age, but chair yoga offers effective strategies to enhance these abilities. By incorporating specific exercises and mindful practices, seniors can improve their ability to focus, retain information, and recall memories more efficiently. These enhancements not only contribute to better daily functioning but also support long-term cognitive health.

One effective method for enhancing memory through chair yoga is Sequential Movement Exercises. These exercises involve performing a series of movements in a specific order, requiring seniors to remember and execute each step accurately. This practice stimulates the brain's memory centers, enhancing both short-term and long-term memory retention. By regularly engaging in sequential movements, individuals can strengthen their ability to remember and recall information, improving overall cognitive function.

Focused Attention Practices are another valuable technique for boosting concentration. These practices involve directing full attention to a single point of focus, such as a specific body part, breath, or movement. By consistently practicing focused attention, seniors can train their minds to maintain concentration for longer periods, reducing susceptibility to distractions. Enhanced concentration not only improves the effectiveness of yoga sessions but also benefits other areas of life that require sustained attention.

Visualization Techniques also play a role in enhancing memory and concentration. By visualizing detailed images or scenarios during yoga practice, seniors engage their imagination and memory simultaneously. This dual engagement strengthens neural pathways associated with both visual memory and cognitive processing, leading to improved recall and mental clarity. Visualization exercises encourage the brain to form vivid, lasting images, which can aid in the retention and retrieval of information.

Additionally, Breathing Exercises for Concentration can significantly enhance cognitive focus. Techniques such as box breathing or alternate nostril breathing require sustained attention to the breath, training the mind to remain present and engaged. These breathing exercises calm the nervous system and sharpen mental focus, making it easier for seniors to concentrate on tasks both during and outside of yoga practice. Improved concentration through breathing exercises contributes to greater mental efficiency and productivity.

Interactive Yoga Sessions that involve memory games or cognitive challenges can further enhance memory and concentration. These sessions might include recalling sequences of movements, repeating mantras, or engaging in dual-task activities that require simultaneous mental and physical engagement. By incorporating these interactive elements, chair yoga becomes a dynamic cognitive workout, stimulating the brain and promoting sustained mental focus. This comprehensive approach ensures that memory and concentration improvements are both significant and long-lasting, supporting overall cognitive health in seniors.

Combining Yoga with Mental Stimulation

Combining yoga with mental stimulation creates a synergistic effect that enhances cognitive functions and promotes overall brain health. For seniors, integrating cognitive challenges with physical movement not only makes yoga sessions more engaging but also supports the maintenance and improvement of various mental abilities. This holistic approach ensures that both the body and mind benefit from the practice, leading to comprehensive well-being.

One effective way to combine yoga with mental stimulation is through Mindful Puzzles and Games During Practice. Incorporating simple puzzles or memory games into yoga sessions encourages seniors to engage their brains while moving. For example, recalling a sequence of poses or solving a riddle before transitioning to the next exercise keeps the mind active and focused. This dual engagement enhances cognitive flexibility and keeps the brain sharp, making the yoga practice both physically and mentally beneficial.

Storytelling and Narrative Techniques can also be integrated into chair yoga to stimulate mental faculties. By weaving stories or guided narratives into yoga sessions, seniors are encouraged to listen, remember, and visualize, which enhances comprehension and memory. This technique transforms yoga into a more interactive and mentally engaging activity, fostering creativity and cognitive engagement. Storytelling within yoga practice not only makes sessions more enjoyable but also promotes deeper mental involvement.

Educational Components can further enrich the combination of yoga and mental stimulation. Including brief educational segments about anatomy, the benefits of specific poses, or the history of yoga can provide cognitive challenges that engage the mind. Learning new information during yoga practice stimulates the brain's learning centers, promoting neural growth and cognitive resilience. This educational approach ensures that seniors are continually exposed to new knowledge, enhancing their intellectual engagement and cognitive health.

Additionally, Mindfulness-Based Cognitive Exercises can be paired with yoga to enhance mental stimulation. These exercises involve techniques such as memory recall, pattern recognition, and problem-solving, integrated seamlessly into yoga routines. For instance, asking participants to recall a sequence of poses or solve a simple puzzle while maintaining their yoga practice engages multiple cognitive domains simultaneously. This multifaceted approach strengthens cognitive abilities and promotes comprehensive mental fitness.

Social Interaction and Group Activities within chair yoga sessions can significantly enhance mental stimulation. Engaging in group discussions, sharing experiences, or participating in cooperative exercises fosters social connections and cognitive engagement. Social interaction stimulates the brain by promoting communication, empathy, and collaborative problem-solving, all of which are essential for maintaining cognitive health. By combining yoga with social and mental activities, seniors can enjoy a more dynamic and mentally enriching practice, supporting both their cognitive and social well-being.

Chapter 13

SPECIALIZED CHAIR YOGA ROUTINES

In this chapter, I will look into a collection of specialized chair yoga routines meticulously designed to address the unique needs and challenges faced by seniors over 70. Understanding that each individual's physical condition and mobility levels vary, I have crafted these routines to offer adaptable and targeted exercises that enhance strength, flexibility, and overall well-being. If you're looking to improve balance, alleviate chronic pain, or simply maintain an active lifestyle, these specialized routines provide the guidance and support necessary to achieve your personal health goals. By incorporating gentle movements, mindful breathing, and thoughtful modifications, I aim to empower you to practice yoga safely and effectively from the comfort of your chair. Join me as we explore these tailored sequences that not only promote physical health but also foster a sense of peace and accomplishment, ensuring that your yoga journey is both enjoyable and beneficial.

Morning Energizer Routine

Wake-Up Stretches

Starting the day with wake-up stretches is essential for seniors to gently awaken the body and prepare it for the activities ahead. These stretches are designed to be performed while seated, ensuring safety and accessibility. Begin by gently tilting your head from side to side, releasing any tension accumulated during sleep. Follow this with shoulder rolls, moving them forward and backward to increase blood flow and reduce stiffness. Neck stretches, such as slowly turning your head to look over each shoulder, help in enhancing flexibility and reducing the risk of strain.

Incorporating arm and wrist stretches can further invigorate the body. Extend your arms forward and interlace your fingers, then gently press your palms away from your body to stretch the forearms. Flexing and extending the wrists in circular motions enhances joint mobility and prepares the upper limbs for the day's activities. Additionally, performing seated torso twists can activate the core muscles, improving posture and encouraging better spinal alignment throughout the day.

Leg stretches are equally important in the morning routine. Begin with seated leg extensions, straightening one leg at a time to engage the quadriceps and hamstrings. Ankle circles and foot flexes promote circulation in the lower limbs, reducing the likelihood of swelling and discomfort. These gentle movements not only enhance flexibility but also contribute to a sense of readiness and alertness.

Incorporating gentle side bends can help in elongating the spine and alleviating any lingering tension in the back and sides of the body. While seated, reach one arm overhead and lean to the opposite side, holding the stretch for a few breaths before switching sides. This movement encourages lateral flexibility and aids in maintaining a healthy range of motion in the spine.

Concluding the wake-up stretches with deep breathing exercises can solidify the benefits of the physical movements. Inhale deeply through the nose, expanding the diaphragm, and exhale slowly through the mouth, releasing any residual tension. This combination of stretching and mindful breathing sets a positive tone for the day, enhancing both physical and mental well-being.

Energizing Breathing Techniques

Breathing techniques play a pivotal role in energizing the body and mind, especially for seniors engaging in chair yoga. One effective method is diaphragmatic breathing, which involves expanding the diaphragm fully while inhaling and contracting it during exhalation. This technique not only increases oxygen intake but also stimulates the parasympathetic nervous system, promoting a sense of calm and focus. To practice, place one hand on the chest and the other on the abdomen, ensuring that only the abdomen rises and falls with each breath.

Another invigorating technique is the "Breath of Fire," a rhythmic and rapid breathing method that enhances energy levels and mental clarity. While seated comfortably, take quick, shallow breaths in and out through the nose, maintaining a steady pace. This technique can be performed for short intervals, gradually increasing the duration as comfort allows. It is important to practice this technique mindfully, avoiding overexertion and ensuring that each breath is controlled and deliberate.

Alternate nostril breathing, or Nadi Shodhana, balances the energy channels in the body and fosters mental equilibrium. Begin by closing the right nostril with the thumb and inhaling deeply through the left nostril. Close the left nostril with the ring finger, release the thumb from the right nostril, and exhale through the right. Inhale through the right nostril, then close it and exhale through the left. This cyclical pattern promotes balance and can be particularly beneficial in reducing anxiety and enhancing concentration.

Box breathing, a structured technique involving equal counts for inhalation, holding, exhalation, and pausing, helps in regulating the breath and calming the mind. For instance, inhale for a count of four, hold the breath for four, exhale for four, and pause for another four counts before repeating. This methodical approach to breathing can enhance focus, reduce stress, and provide a sense of stability, making it an excellent addition to the morning routine.

Integrating these energizing breathing techniques with the physical movements of chair yoga creates a harmonious blend of body and mind stimulation. Practicing them regularly can lead to improved respiratory function, increased energy levels, and a heightened sense of awareness. Seniors can adapt these techniques to their comfort levels, ensuring that each breath is both purposeful and beneficial.

Gentle Movement to Start the Day

Incorporating gentle movements into the morning routine helps in gradually waking up the muscles and joints, fostering a sense of vitality and readiness for the day. One such movement is seated marching, where seniors lift one knee at a time in a controlled manner, mimicking the action of marching. This exercise promotes circulation in the lower body and engages the core muscles, enhancing overall stability and coordination.

Another beneficial movement is the seated cat-cow stretch, adapted from traditional yoga poses to be performed while sitting. By alternately arching the back and rounding the spine, seniors can improve spinal flexibility and relieve tension in the back and neck. This fluid motion not only enhances mobility but also encourages mindful movement, connecting breath with each motion to maximize the benefits.

Seated side leg lifts are also effective in activating the lower body muscles without putting undue strain on the joints. By lifting one leg to the side while keeping the core engaged, seniors can strengthen the hip abductors and improve balance. This movement can be performed slowly and deliberately, ensuring that each lift is controlled and supported by the chair.

Incorporating gentle arm circles into the morning routine can further energize the upper body. By extending the arms to the sides and making small, controlled circles, seniors can enhance shoulder mobility and increase blood flow to the upper limbs. This simple yet effective movement helps in reducing stiffness and preparing the arms for daily activities.

Integrating seated spinal twists into the morning movement sequence encourages rotational flexibility and engages the abdominal muscles. By twisting the torso gently to one side and then the other, seniors can improve spinal health and stimulate the digestive system. This movement not only contributes to physical flexibility but also fosters a sense of mental clarity and readiness to embrace the day ahead.

Evening Relaxation Routine

Calming Stretches

As the day winds down, engaging in calming stretches can help seniors release the accumulated tension and prepare the body for restful sleep. Beginning with gentle neck stretches, seniors can slowly tilt their heads forward, backward, and side to side, easing any stiffness and promoting relaxation. These movements should be performed slowly and mindfully, ensuring that each stretch is held for several breaths to maximize the calming effects.

Incorporating seated forward bends into the evening routine can further enhance relaxation. By reaching towards the toes while keeping the spine elongated, seniors can stretch the lower back and hamstrings, alleviating any discomfort from prolonged sitting or activity. This forward movement encourages the release of built-up tension and promotes a sense of calmness in the body.

Arm and shoulder stretches are also crucial in the evening routine. Seniors can extend one arm across the chest and gently press it with the opposite hand, stretching the shoulder muscles and relieving any tightness from the day's activities. Additionally, overhead arm stretches, where arms are lifted and gently pulled back, can open up the chest and improve upper body flexibility, contributing to overall relaxation.

Seated spinal twists can be revisited in the evening to further aid in releasing tension from the back and spine. By twisting the torso gently to each side, seniors can massage the internal organs and improve digestion, which is beneficial before bedtime. This movement also helps in winding down the nervous system, preparing the body for a restful night.

Concluding the calming stretches with gentle ankle and wrist rotations ensures that all joints are relaxed and free from tension. By slowly rotating the ankles and wrists in circular motions, seniors can enhance joint mobility and promote a sense of completeness in the relaxation routine. These final stretches help in calming the entire body, setting the stage for a peaceful transition to sleep.

Evening Meditation Practices

Evening meditation practices are integral to the relaxation routine, offering seniors a way to unwind mentally and emotionally before bedtime. One effective practice is guided visualization, where seniors are encouraged to imagine serene and peaceful settings, such as a quiet beach or a tranquil garden. This mental imagery helps in diverting the mind from daily stresses and fosters a sense of inner peace and tranquility.

Another valuable meditation technique is progressive muscle relaxation, which involves systematically tensing and then relaxing different muscle groups. Starting from the feet and moving upwards, seniors can focus on each part of the body, releasing any residual tension and promoting overall relaxation. This method not only aids in physical relaxation but also enhances body awareness and mindfulness.

Breath-focused meditation is also beneficial in the evening routine. By concentrating solely on the breath, seniors can anchor their minds and cultivate a sense of presence. Simple practices, such as counting breaths or repeating a calming mantra, can help in quieting the mind and preparing it for restful sleep. This focus on breathing promotes deep relaxation and reduces anxiety, making it easier to drift into sleep.

Mindfulness meditation, which emphasizes being present in the moment without judgment, can further enhance the evening relaxation routine. Seniors can practice mindfulness by paying attention to sensory experiences, such as the feeling of the chair beneath them or the sounds in their environment. This heightened awareness fosters a deep sense of calm and can improve overall mental well-being.

Concluding the meditation practice with a few moments of silent reflection allows seniors to internalize the benefits of their practice. By sitting quietly and embracing the stillness, they can cultivate a peaceful state of mind, ready to transition into a restful night's sleep. This silent reflection reinforces the day's positive experiences and sets a positive tone for the following day.

Preparing the Body for Rest

Preparing the body for rest through specific chair yoga movements can significantly improve sleep quality and overall well-being for seniors. Gentle stretches aimed at releasing tension from the back and shoulders are particularly effective. By performing slow shoulder shrugs and rolls, seniors can alleviate any stiffness and promote relaxation in the upper body, making it easier to settle into a restful state.

Leg stretches designed for the evening routine can help in reducing any residual fatigue in the lower limbs. Seated hamstring stretches, where one leg is extended while keeping the back straight, can ease tension in the legs and lower back. Additionally, gentle calf raises and seated toe taps can promote blood circulation and prevent any discomfort during sleep.

Incorporating deep breathing exercises into the evening routine is crucial for preparing the body for rest. By practicing slow, deep breaths, seniors can activate the body's relaxation response, lowering heart rate and reducing stress levels. This mindful breathing helps in calming the nervous system and creating a conducive environment for sleep.

Seated forward bends and gentle twists can further prepare the body for rest by promoting spinal alignment and releasing any remaining tension. These movements encourage the flow of energy throughout the body, aiding in the detoxification process and enhancing overall relaxation. By aligning the spine and releasing muscular tension, seniors can create a sense of harmony and balance in their bodies.

Concluding the evening routine with a brief period of silent meditation or reflection allows seniors to fully embrace the relaxation achieved through their chair yoga practice. This final step reinforces the body's readiness for rest, ensuring that both the mind and body are prepared for a night of restorative sleep. By consistently following this routine, seniors can experience improved sleep quality and enhanced overall health.

Therapeutic Yoga for Specific Conditions

Diabetes Management

Chair yoga can play a supportive role in managing diabetes by promoting overall health and well-being. Engaging in regular chair yoga sessions helps in improving blood circulation, which is crucial for individuals with diabetes. Enhanced circulation can aid in the effective distribution of insulin and nutrients throughout the body, contributing to better blood sugar regulation. Additionally, the gentle movements involved in chair yoga help in reducing stress, which is known to impact blood glucose levels negatively.

Incorporating specific poses that target the lower body can be particularly beneficial for diabetes management. Seated leg lifts and ankle rotations improve blood flow to the extremities, reducing the risk of complications such as peripheral neuropathy. Strengthening the lower body muscles through chair yoga can also enhance insulin sensitivity, making the body's cells more responsive to insulin and aiding in more efficient glucose uptake.

Breathing techniques practiced during chair yoga can help in managing stress and anxiety, common issues faced by individuals with diabetes. Deep breathing exercises, such as diaphragmatic breathing, activate the parasympathetic nervous system, promoting relaxation and reducing cortisol levels. Lower stress levels contribute to better blood sugar control and overall health, making these techniques an integral part of diabetes management.

Mindfulness meditation, incorporated into the chair yoga routine, encourages individuals to develop a greater awareness of their bodies and health. This heightened awareness can lead to better self-management of diabetes, as individuals become more attuned to their body's signals and needs. Mindfulness practices also foster a positive mindset, which can enhance adherence to diabetes treatment plans and lifestyle modifications.

Chair yoga supports weight management, a key factor in diabetes control. By engaging in regular physical activity through chair yoga, individuals can maintain a healthy weight, reducing the risk of insulin resistance and improving overall metabolic health. Combined with mindful eating and nutritional guidance, chair yoga becomes a holistic approach to managing diabetes, enhancing both physical and mental well-being.

Heart Health Focus

Chair yoga offers numerous benefits for heart health, making it a valuable practice for seniors concerned about cardiovascular well-being. Regular engagement in chair yoga can help in lowering blood pressure, a significant risk factor for heart disease. The gentle movements and deep breathing techniques employed in chair yoga promote relaxation and reduce stress, both of which contribute to healthier blood pressure levels.

Incorporating poses that enhance circulation is particularly beneficial for heart health. Seated forward bends and gentle twists encourage blood flow to the heart and vital organs, ensuring that the body receives adequate oxygen and nutrients. Improved circulation also aids in the removal of metabolic waste products, supporting overall cardiovascular function.

Strengthening the upper body through chair yoga can have a positive impact on heart health. Exercises such as seated arm raises and shoulder presses enhance muscle tone and endurance, promoting a more efficient heart. A stronger upper body requires less effort from the heart during daily activities, reducing the overall workload on the cardiovascular system and contributing to better heart health.

Breathing exercises integral to chair yoga play a crucial role in managing heart rate and reducing cardiac stress. Techniques like alternate nostril breathing and deep diaphragmatic breathing help in regulating heart rate variability, promoting a balanced and steady heartbeat. These breathing practices not only enhance oxygenation but also foster a sense of calm, mitigating the effects of stress on the heart.

The meditative aspects of chair yoga contribute to emotional well-being, which is intrinsically linked to heart health. By fostering mindfulness and reducing anxiety, chair yoga helps in maintaining a positive mental state, which is essential for cardiovascular health. A balanced and peaceful mind supports healthy heart function, making chair yoga a comprehensive approach to promoting heart health in seniors.

Respiratory Support Exercises

Chair yoga includes various respiratory support exercises that can significantly benefit seniors by enhancing lung capacity and improving overall respiratory function. One fundamental technique is diaphragmatic breathing, which emphasizes deep, abdominal breaths that fully engage the diaphragm. This method increases oxygen intake and strengthens the respiratory muscles, making breathing more efficient and reducing the effort required for each breath.

Incorporating pranayama, or breath control exercises, into the chair yoga routine can further support respiratory health. Practices such as alternate nostril breathing and ujjayi breath (victorious breath) help in regulating the breath and enhancing lung function. These techniques promote better airflow, reduce respiratory fatigue, and improve the body's ability to utilize oxygen effectively.

Seated thoracic expansions are another valuable exercise for respiratory support. By gently arching the back and expanding the chest while inhaling, seniors can increase the flexibility of the ribcage and improve lung expansion. This movement facilitates deeper breaths and enhances the overall capacity of the lungs, making it easier to breathe comfortably throughout the day.

Incorporating gentle side stretches into the routine can also aid in respiratory support. By extending the arms overhead and leaning to one side, seniors can create more space in the chest cavity, allowing for greater lung expansion. These side stretches not only improve flexibility but also enhance the efficiency of the respiratory system, contributing to better overall lung health.

Integrating relaxation techniques with respiratory support exercises can optimize the benefits for seniors. By combining deep breathing with guided relaxation or visualization, chair yoga helps in reducing respiratory rate and promoting a state of calm. This holistic approach ensures that the respiratory system is not only strengthened but also harmonized with the body's natural rhythms, fostering long-term respiratory health and well-being.

Chapter 14

INTEGRATING YOGA INTO DAILY LIFE

I believe that the true essence of yoga lies not just in the exercises themselves, but in seamlessly weaving these practices into the fabric of our everyday routines. Throughout my years of teaching and practicing yoga with seniors, I have witnessed firsthand how integrating simple yoga techniques into daily activities can transform lives, enhancing both physical health and mental well-being. In this chapter, I share practical strategies and personal insights on how to make yoga a natural and enjoyable part of your day, whether you're starting with morning stretches to greet the day, incorporating mindful breathing during meals, or unwinding with gentle poses before bedtime. By embracing these small, consistent practices, you can cultivate a sustainable yoga habit that supports your journey towards greater flexibility, strength, and inner peace. My goal is to empower you to create a personalized yoga routine that fits effortlessly into your lifestyle, making the benefits of yoga accessible and enduring for years to come.

Creating a Daily Yoga Schedule

Setting Consistent Times for Practice

Establishing a consistent time for your daily yoga practice is essential for building a sustainable routine. By selecting specific times each day, you create a sense of structure that can help reinforce the habit of practicing chair yoga. Whether you choose to begin your day with morning stretches or wind down in the evening with relaxation techniques, consistency ensures that yoga becomes an integral part of your daily life rather than an occasional activity.

Morning sessions can invigorate your body and mind, setting a positive tone for the rest of the day. Starting with gentle stretches can help awaken your muscles, improve circulation, and enhance mental clarity, preparing you for the activities ahead. Alternatively, evening practices can aid in unwinding, reducing stress accumulated throughout the day, and promoting restful sleep. The key is to identify the time that best aligns with your personal energy levels and daily commitments.

Creating a consistent schedule also helps in tracking your progress and maintaining motivation. When yoga becomes a regular part of your day, you're more likely to notice improvements in flexibility, strength, and overall well-being. Keeping a yoga journal can complement your schedule, allowing you to document your experiences, set goals, and reflect on your journey. This practice not only reinforces your commitment but also provides a sense of accomplishment as you observe your growth over time.

Flexibility within your schedule is equally important. Life can be unpredictable, and having the ability to adjust your practice times without feeling discouraged ensures that yoga remains a positive and enjoyable experience. If morning sessions become challenging due to unforeseen circumstances, having an alternative time slot can help you stay on track without added stress. The objective is to make yoga a flexible yet consistent part of your lifestyle.

Setting reminders can be a practical tool in maintaining your yoga schedule. Utilizing alarms, calendar notifications, or even visual cues around your living space can prompt you to engage in your practice regularly. These reminders serve as gentle nudges, ensuring that yoga remains a priority amidst the demands of daily life. By integrating these strategies, you can establish a reliable and fulfilling daily yoga routine that enhances your overall well-being.

Balancing Yoga with Other Activities

Balancing yoga with other daily activities requires thoughtful planning and prioritization. As you incorporate chair yoga into your routine, it's important to ensure that it complements rather than disrupts your existing commitments. This balance can be achieved by aligning your yoga sessions with other activities that promote health and well-being, creating a harmonious blend of physical and mental practices.

One effective strategy is to integrate yoga into transitional periods of your day. For example, practicing yoga after a meal can aid digestion and prevent the lethargy that often follows eating. Similarly, incorporating short yoga breaks between tasks can rejuvenate your mind and body, enhancing productivity and focus. By strategically placing yoga sessions within your daily schedule, you can maintain a balanced approach that supports your overall lifestyle.

Another aspect of balancing yoga with other activities involves understanding your personal energy levels and preferences. Some individuals may find that yoga energizes them, making it a perfect fit for morning routines, while others might prefer the calming effects of yoga in the evening to wind down. Listening to your body's needs and adjusting your yoga practice accordingly ensures that it enhances rather than competes with your daily activities.

Moreover, integrating yoga with other forms of exercise or hobbies can create a well-rounded approach to health and wellness. Combining chair yoga with activities such as walking, gardening, or light strength training can provide comprehensive benefits, addressing different aspects of physical fitness. This combination not only prevents monotony but also ensures that various muscle groups are engaged, promoting overall physical harmony.

Finally, maintaining flexibility in your schedule allows for adjustments as needed. Life's unpredictability means that some days may require rearranging your activities to accommodate unforeseen events. Being adaptable ensures that yoga remains a positive and manageable part of your routine, without causing undue stress or imbalance. By embracing flexibility and thoughtful planning, you can successfully balance yoga with other essential activities, fostering a holistic and fulfilling lifestyle.

Adapting to Changing Schedules

As life evolves, so too will your daily schedule. Adapting your yoga practice to accommodate changes in your routine is crucial for maintaining consistency and reaping the benefits of chair yoga over the long term. Whether due to seasonal shifts, health considerations, or alterations in personal commitments, being adaptable ensures that yoga remains a steadfast component of your wellness regimen.

One effective approach to adapting your yoga schedule is to reassess and realign your priorities regularly. Periodic evaluations of your daily activities and energy levels can help you identify the most suitable times for practice. For instance, during winter months when daylight hours are shorter, you might find it beneficial to shift your yoga sessions to earlier in the day. Similarly, during periods of increased social or family commitments, adjusting the duration or frequency of your practice can help maintain balance.

Incorporating flexibility into your yoga routine also involves modifying the intensity and duration of your sessions based on your current physical condition. Health fluctuations, such as minor illnesses or increased fatigue, may necessitate gentler stretches or shorter practice periods. Being mindful of your body's signals and adjusting your practice accordingly ensures that yoga remains a supportive and non-strenuous activity, promoting sustained well-being without causing strain.

Technology can also play a pivotal role in adapting your yoga schedule. Utilizing digital tools such as yoga apps, online classes, or virtual reminders can provide the flexibility needed to practice anytime and anywhere. These resources offer a variety of routines and modifications, allowing you to tailor your practice to fit seamlessly into changing schedules. Additionally, virtual communities can offer support and motivation, helping you stay committed despite external changes.

Maintaining a positive and resilient mindset is essential when adapting to schedule changes. Embracing flexibility as a natural part of life rather than viewing it as a challenge can transform your approach to yoga practice. Recognizing that adjustments are necessary for sustained health and well-being allows you to remain committed to your practice, even when faced with unforeseen circumstances. By fostering adaptability, you ensure that chair yoga continues to enhance your daily life, regardless of the changes that may arise.

Yoga for Everyday Activities

Enhancing Mobility for Daily Tasks

Enhancing mobility through chair yoga can significantly improve your ability to perform daily tasks with greater ease and comfort. As we age, maintaining flexibility and joint health becomes increasingly important to support independence and quality of life. Chair yoga offers a gentle yet effective means of promoting mobility, enabling seniors to engage in everyday activities without undue strain or discomfort.

Daily tasks such as reaching for items, bending, or standing can become challenging due to decreased mobility. Incorporating specific chair yoga exercises can target the muscles and joints involved in these movements, enhancing their range of motion and reducing stiffness. For example, seated leg lifts and ankle rotations can improve lower body flexibility, making tasks like walking or climbing stairs more manageable.

Moreover, enhanced mobility contributes to better posture and balance, which are crucial for preventing falls and injuries. Strengthening the core and back muscles through chair yoga can provide the necessary support for maintaining an upright posture, reducing the risk of slouching or leaning excessively. Improved balance, achieved through targeted exercises, ensures greater stability during daily movements, fostering confidence and safety.

In addition to physical benefits, increased mobility has positive effects on mental and emotional well-being. Being able to move freely and perform tasks independently fosters a sense of accomplishment and self-sufficiency, boosting self-esteem and reducing feelings of frustration or helplessness. This enhanced sense of control over one's body and environment contributes to overall happiness and life satisfaction.

Integrating mobility-enhancing yoga exercises into your daily routine can lead to long-term benefits that extend beyond physical capabilities. As mobility improves, you may find yourself more inclined to participate in various activities, social engagements, and hobbies that were previously limited by physical constraints. This expanded range of experiences not only enriches your life but also promotes continued physical and mental health through active engagement.

Incorporating Stretching into Routine Chores

Incorporating stretching exercises into your routine chores is a practical way to blend physical activity with everyday responsibilities. This approach not only maximizes time efficiency but also ensures that you maintain flexibility and strength throughout the day. By integrating chair yoga stretches into tasks such as cooking, cleaning, or organizing, you create a seamless flow between productivity and wellness.

For instance, while waiting for water to boil or during cooking preparations, you can perform gentle neck and shoulder stretches to alleviate tension accumulated from standing or repetitive movements. Similarly, during cleaning activities like dusting or wiping surfaces, incorporating arm and wrist stretches can prevent strain and enhance endurance. These simple additions transform mundane chores into opportunities for maintaining physical health.

Moreover, combining stretching with routine chores promotes consistency in your yoga practice. As you associate specific tasks with particular stretches, you create habitual triggers that remind you to engage in physical activity regularly. This habitual integration ensures that stretching becomes a natural part of your day, reducing the likelihood of neglecting your yoga practice amidst other responsibilities.

In addition to physical benefits, incorporating stretching into routine chores can enhance mental focus and mindfulness. Engaging in mindful stretching while performing tasks encourages a state of present awareness, reducing stress and promoting mental clarity. This dual focus on physical movement and mental presence enriches the overall experience, making everyday activities more enjoyable and less burdensome.

Adapting your environment to support integrated stretching can further facilitate this practice. Ensuring that your living space is organized and accessible allows for smoother transitions between chores and stretching exercises. For example, positioning a comfortable chair in your kitchen or living area provides a convenient spot for performing seated stretches without disrupting your workflow. By thoughtfully incorporating stretching into routine chores, you cultivate a balanced and health-conscious lifestyle that seamlessly blends productivity with well-being.

Using Yoga to Improve Daily Comfort

Using yoga to improve daily comfort involves integrating mindful movements and postures that alleviate common discomforts and enhance overall physical ease. Chair yoga offers a range of exercises tailored to address specific areas of tension and pain, making it an invaluable tool for seniors seeking to enhance their daily comfort. By focusing on gentle stretches and strengthening exercises, chair yoga can transform your daily experience, making everyday activities more pleasant and less taxing on the body.

One common source of discomfort among seniors is back pain, often resulting from prolonged sitting or poor posture. Incorporating seated spinal twists and gentle forward bends can help alleviate back tension, promote spinal flexibility, and reduce pain. These exercises not only relieve immediate discomfort but also contribute to long-term spinal health, making it easier to maintain an upright and comfortable posture throughout the day.

Neck and shoulder stiffness, frequently caused by activities such as reading or using electronic devices, can also be mitigated through targeted yoga movements. Simple neck stretches and shoulder rolls can increase blood flow, reduce muscle tightness, and enhance range of motion. These practices ensure that your upper body remains relaxed and flexible, preventing the buildup of tension that can lead to chronic pain and discomfort.

Incorporating yoga into your daily routine can also improve circulation and reduce swelling in the extremities. Seated leg lifts, ankle circles, and gentle foot stretches promote blood flow, preventing issues such as varicose veins or edema. Enhanced circulation not only reduces physical discomfort but also boosts overall vitality, making you feel more energized and comfortable throughout the day.

Additionally, chair yoga fosters a sense of relaxation and mental ease, which directly contributes to daily comfort. Engaging in breathing exercises and mindfulness practices can alleviate stress and anxiety, promoting a calm and balanced mental state. This mental relaxation complements the physical benefits of yoga, ensuring that you experience a holistic improvement in comfort and well-being as you navigate your daily activities.

Building a Supportive Community

Joining Chair Yoga Classes

Joining chair yoga classes is an excellent way to enhance your practice and connect with others who share similar wellness goals. These classes provide structured guidance from experienced instructors who understand the unique needs and limitations of seniors. Participating in a class setting offers a supportive environment where you can learn new techniques, receive personalized feedback, and stay motivated through group encouragement.

Attending chair yoga classes, whether in-person or virtual, introduces you to a community of peers who can offer companionship and mutual support. This social aspect is particularly beneficial for seniors, as it fosters a sense of belonging and reduces feelings of isolation.

Engaging with others in a shared activity creates opportunities for meaningful interactions and friendships, enhancing both your physical and emotional well-being.

Instructors in chair yoga classes are trained to modify poses and adapt routines to accommodate varying levels of ability and fitness. This personalized approach ensures that each participant can practice safely and effectively, addressing their specific needs and limitations. Through regular participation, you can develop a deeper understanding of your body, refine your techniques, and progress at a comfortable pace under professional supervision.

Moreover, joining a class provides access to a variety of yoga styles and routines, broadening your practice and preventing monotony. Exposure to different sequences and exercises keeps your sessions engaging and challenging, promoting continuous improvement and sustained interest. This diversity in practice enhances your overall flexibility, strength, and mobility, contributing to a well-rounded yoga experience.

Chair yoga classes often incorporate elements of mindfulness and meditation, enriching your practice beyond physical exercise. These sessions guide you in cultivating mental clarity, reducing stress, and enhancing emotional resilience. By joining chair yoga classes, you not only improve your physical health but also nurture your mental and emotional well-being, achieving a holistic approach to wellness within a supportive community framework.

Engaging with Online Yoga Communities

Engaging with online yoga communities offers a flexible and accessible way to enhance your chair yoga practice from the comfort of your home. These virtual communities provide a platform for sharing experiences, exchanging tips, and receiving encouragement from fellow practitioners around the world. Participating in online forums, social media groups, or virtual classes can significantly enrich your yoga journey, offering a sense of connection and support regardless of geographical limitations.

Online yoga communities often feature a wealth of resources, including instructional videos, live classes, and interactive webinars led by experienced instructors. These resources allow you to explore various aspects of chair yoga at your own pace, enabling you to tailor your practice to your specific needs and preferences. Access to diverse content ensures that your practice remains dynamic and adaptable, fostering continuous growth and improvement.

Additionally, online communities provide opportunities for personalized feedback and guidance. Through live interactions, you can receive real-time corrections and suggestions from instructors, enhancing the effectiveness and safety of your practice. Engaging in Q&A sessions or seeking advice on specific challenges allows you to address individual concerns and refine your techniques, promoting a more effective and fulfilling yoga experience.

Moreover, participating in online challenges or group practices can boost your motivation and commitment to regular yoga sessions. These communal activities create a sense of accountability, encouraging you to stay consistent with your practice. Celebrating milestones and achievements within the community fosters a positive and encouraging environment, reinforcing your dedication and inspiring others to pursue their wellness goals.

Online yoga communities facilitate the sharing of personal stories and experiences, creating a supportive network where members can uplift and inspire each other. Hearing about others' journeys, overcoming obstacles, and celebrating successes can provide valuable insights and encouragement. This shared sense of purpose and camaraderie enhances your overall experience, making your chair yoga practice more enjoyable and deeply integrated into your daily life.

Sharing Progress with Friends and Family

Sharing your yoga progress with friends and family can significantly enhance your motivation and sense of achievement. Communicating your goals, milestones, and experiences with loved ones fosters a supportive environment that encourages continued commitment to your practice. This openness not only strengthens your relationships but also provides additional accountability, making it easier to stay dedicated to your wellness journey.

When you share your progress, you invite others to celebrate your successes and offer encouragement during challenging times. This emotional support can be invaluable, especially when faced with setbacks or difficulties in your practice. Friends and family can provide positive reinforcement, helping you maintain a positive mindset and stay focused on your goals. Their encouragement acts as a motivational boost, inspiring you to persevere and continue striving for improvement.

Moreover, involving loved ones in your yoga practice can create shared experiences that strengthen bonds and foster mutual understanding. Encouraging a family member or friend to join you in chair yoga sessions can turn your practice into a collaborative and enjoyable activity. This shared commitment not only enhances your practice but also creates opportunities for quality time and meaningful connections, enriching your social life alongside your physical health.

Sharing your journey can also inspire others to embark on their own wellness paths. By openly discussing the benefits you've experienced and the progress you've made, you can motivate those around you to explore chair yoga or other forms of exercise. Your story serves as a testament to the positive impact of yoga, encouraging others to prioritize their health and well-being, thereby creating a ripple effect of wellness within your community.

Chapter 15

MAINTAINING LONG-TERM WELLNESS

Maintaining long-term wellness through chair yoga involves more than just performing regular exercises. It encompasses tracking your progress, adapting your practice as your needs evolve, and staying motivated to continue your journey toward better health and well-being. This chapter provides strategies and insights to help you sustain and enhance the benefits you have gained from chair yoga over time.

Tracking Your Progress

1. Journaling Your Yoga Journey

Journaling your yoga journey is a powerful tool for tracking progress and reflecting on your personal growth. By maintaining a dedicated yoga journal, you can document each session, noting the poses practiced, durations, and any challenges faced. This record serves as a tangible reminder of your commitment and the consistency of your practice. Additionally, journaling allows you to identify patterns in your physical and mental states, helping you understand how yoga positively impacts your daily life.

Beyond tracking physical exercises, a yoga journal can capture your emotional and mental experiences. Writing about your feelings before and after each session can highlight the stress-relief and mental clarity benefits of yoga. Over time, these entries can reveal significant improvements in your mood, cognitive function, and overall sense of well-being. This reflective practice encourages mindfulness and reinforces the connection between your mind and body.

Moreover, journaling fosters accountability. By setting aside a few minutes after each session to record your experiences, you create a routine that reinforces your commitment to yoga. This habit can be particularly beneficial during times when motivation wanes, serving as a motivational tool to remind you of your progress and the positive changes you have achieved.

In addition to personal reflection, your yoga journal can be a valuable resource when consulting with healthcare professionals or yoga instructors. Detailed records of your practice can provide insights into your physical capabilities and any areas that may require additional attention or modification. This information can guide personalized adjustments to your yoga routines, ensuring that your practice remains safe and effective.

Revisiting past journal entries can be incredibly inspiring. Seeing how far you have come can boost your confidence and encourage you to set new goals. It also serves as a reminder of the resilience and dedication you have demonstrated throughout your yoga journey, reinforcing the importance of maintaining long-term wellness through consistent practice.

2. Setting and Reviewing Goals

Setting clear and achievable goals is essential for maintaining long-term wellness through chair yoga. Goals provide direction and purpose, helping you stay focused and motivated. Begin by identifying both short-term and long-term objectives that align with your personal health and wellness aspirations. Short-term goals might include mastering a particular pose or increasing the duration of your practice, while long-term goals could involve significant improvements in flexibility, strength, or overall health.

When setting goals, it is important to make them specific, measurable, attainable, relevant, and time-bound (SMART). For example, instead of setting a vague goal like "improve flexibility," a SMART goal would be "increase the range of motion in my shoulders by practicing specific stretches three times a week for the next two months." This approach ensures that your goals are clear and achievable, providing a structured path to follow.

Regularly reviewing your goals is just as crucial as setting them. Schedule periodic check-ins to assess your progress and determine whether adjustments are needed. This practice allows you to celebrate your achievements and recognize areas where you may need to refocus your efforts. It also provides an opportunity to set new goals as you reach previous milestones, ensuring that your practice continues to evolve and challenge you.

Incorporating flexibility into your goal-setting process is important, especially as your physical capabilities and health needs change over time. Be prepared to modify your goals based on your progress and any new insights you gain from your practice. This adaptability ensures that your goals remain relevant and attainable, preventing frustration and promoting sustained engagement with your yoga routine.

Sharing your goals with a trusted friend, family member, or yoga instructor can provide additional support and accountability. Discussing your objectives can offer new perspectives and encouragement, making it easier to stay committed to your long-term wellness journey. Collaborative goal-setting can also introduce new ideas and strategies, enriching your practice and enhancing your overall experience with chair yoga.

3. Celebrating Milestones and Achievements

Celebrating milestones and achievements is a vital component of maintaining long-term wellness through chair yoga. Recognizing and honoring your progress reinforces positive behavior and keeps you motivated to continue your practice. Milestones can be as simple as completing your first week of consistent yoga sessions or as significant as achieving a major flexibility or strength goal. Celebrating these achievements acknowledges your hard work and dedication, providing a sense of accomplishment that fuels ongoing commitment.

One effective way to celebrate milestones is by setting up small rewards for yourself. These rewards can range from enjoying a favorite healthy treat, purchasing new yoga accessories, or dedicating time to a leisure activity you enjoy. Rewards serve as incentives that make reaching your goals more enjoyable and provide tangible acknowledgment of your efforts. They also help create positive associations with your yoga practice, making it a source of joy and satisfaction.

In addition to personal rewards, sharing your achievements with others can enhance the celebration. Communicating your progress with friends, family, or fellow yoga practitioners can provide a sense of community and support. Their encouragement and recognition can boost your confidence and inspire you to set and pursue new goals. Social acknowledgment of your achievements can also foster a sense of belonging, making your yoga journey a shared and enriching experience.

Another meaningful way to celebrate milestones is by reflecting on your journey and documenting your progress. Creating a visual representation of your achievements, such as a progress chart or a photo diary, can offer a tangible record of your growth. This reflection not only highlights your successes but also reinforces the positive changes you have experienced through yoga. It serves as a powerful reminder of your resilience and the benefits of maintaining a consistent practice.

Celebrating milestones encourages a positive mindset and fosters a sense of gratitude. Acknowledging your achievements helps you appreciate the journey and the efforts you have invested in your health and well-being. This positive outlook can enhance your overall quality of life, making it easier to stay motivated and committed to your long-term wellness goals. By celebrating your milestones, you honor your journey and inspire yourself to continue striving for better health and happiness through chair yoga.

Adapting Your Practice Over Time

1. Modifying Exercises as Needs Change

As we age, our bodies undergo various changes that can affect our physical capabilities and health needs. It is essential to adapt your chair yoga practice to accommodate these changes, ensuring that your exercises remain safe, effective, and enjoyable. Modifying poses and routines can help address specific health concerns, such as joint pain or reduced mobility, while still allowing you to reap the benefits of yoga. This adaptability ensures that your practice evolves in harmony with your body's needs, promoting sustained wellness.

One common modification involves adjusting the intensity and duration of exercises. If you experience increased stiffness or fatigue, reducing the number of repetitions or the time spent in each pose can prevent overexertion and reduce the risk of injury. Additionally, incorporating more frequent breaks and focusing on gentle movements can make your practice more comfortable and accessible. Listening to your body and making these adjustments ensures that your yoga sessions remain enjoyable and beneficial.

Another way to modify your practice is by utilizing supportive props and equipment. Items such as resistance bands, cushions, or yoga straps can provide additional support and stability, making certain poses easier to perform. For instance, using a cushion under your back can enhance comfort during seated poses, while resistance bands can assist in strength-building exercises. These tools allow you to customize your practice, ensuring that each exercise aligns with your current physical condition.

Incorporating alternative poses is also an effective strategy for adapting your practice. If a particular pose becomes challenging or uncomfortable, replacing it with a similar alternative can maintain the benefits without causing strain. For example, if a seated twist becomes too difficult, opting for a simpler side stretch can still enhance flexibility and mobility. Exploring different variations of poses ensures that your practice remains dynamic and responsive to your body's evolving needs.

Consulting with healthcare professionals or experienced yoga instructors can provide valuable insights into modifying your practice. These experts can offer personalized recommendations based on your health status and fitness level, ensuring that your exercises are both safe and effective. Regularly updating your practice with professional guidance helps you stay aligned with your wellness goals and maintain a healthy, balanced approach to chair yoga.

2. Exploring Advanced Chair Yoga Techniques

As you become more comfortable and proficient with chair yoga, you may find yourself ready to explore advanced techniques that further enhance your practice. Advanced chair yoga can introduce new challenges and opportunities for growth, allowing you to deepen your physical and mental engagement. These techniques can include more complex poses, extended sequences, and integrated mindfulness practices that elevate your overall yoga experience.

One advanced technique involves incorporating dynamic movements and transitions between poses. Flowing smoothly from one pose to another can increase the intensity of your workout, promoting greater flexibility and cardiovascular health. For example, transitioning from a seated forward bend to a gentle twist can create a fluid sequence that engages multiple muscle groups and enhances coordination. These dynamic sequences keep your practice varied and stimulating, preventing monotony and maintaining your interest.

Another advanced approach is the integration of strength-building exercises with traditional yoga poses. Adding resistance through the use of weights or resistance bands can amplify the benefits of your practice, contributing to increased muscle tone and endurance. For instance, performing seated bicep curls with light weights while holding a steady pose can simultaneously strengthen your arms and improve your balance. These combined exercises provide a more comprehensive workout, supporting overall physical health.

Incorporating deeper mindfulness and meditation practices can also elevate your chair yoga experience. Advanced meditation techniques, such as guided visualizations or focused breathing exercises, can enhance your mental clarity and emotional resilience. By dedicating more time to mindfulness, you can cultivate a greater sense of inner peace and presence, complementing the physical benefits of yoga. These practices foster a holistic approach to wellness, addressing both body and mind.

Exploring thematic yoga sessions can add variety and purpose to your advanced practice. Themes such as gratitude, relaxation, or vitality can guide your choice of poses and meditation focus, creating a more meaningful and personalized experience. For example, a gratitude-themed session might include poses that open the heart and promote a sense of thankfulness, while a vitality-themed session could emphasize energizing movements and invigorating breathwork. These thematic approaches enrich your practice, making each session uniquely fulfilling and aligned with your personal growth.

3. Staying Motivated for Continued Growth

Staying motivated is crucial for maintaining a long-term chair yoga practice, especially as initial enthusiasm may wane over time. Developing strategies to keep your motivation high ensures that you continue to prioritize your wellness and reap the ongoing benefits of yoga. Motivation can be sustained through a combination of goal-setting, variety in your practice, community support, and personal rewards that celebrate your dedication and progress.

One effective way to maintain motivation is by regularly setting new and diverse goals. As you achieve initial objectives, establishing new ones keeps your practice challenging and engaging. These goals can range from mastering specific poses to increasing the duration of your sessions or exploring new yoga techniques. Continuously striving for improvement provides a sense of purpose and accomplishment, driving you to remain committed to your yoga routine.

Incorporating variety into your practice can also help sustain your interest and enthusiasm. Exploring different styles of chair yoga, trying new sequences, or integrating different mindfulness practices can prevent your routine from becoming monotonous. Variety not only keeps your sessions fresh and exciting but also ensures that you are continuously stimulating different muscle groups and aspects of your mental well-being. This dynamic approach enhances the overall effectiveness of your practice and keeps you engaged.

Engaging with a supportive community can significantly boost your motivation. Participating in group classes, either in person or online, allows you to connect with fellow practitioners who share similar goals and challenges. Sharing experiences, offering encouragement, and celebrating each other's successes fosters a sense of camaraderie and accountability. This communal support can be a powerful motivator, reminding you that you are part of a larger network committed to wellness and growth.

Additionally, recognizing and rewarding your achievements plays a vital role in maintaining motivation. Celebrating milestones, no matter how small, reinforces your commitment and provides positive reinforcement for your efforts. Rewards can be simple, such as treating yourself to a favorite activity, purchasing new yoga equipment, or enjoying a special meal. These incentives make your achievements more tangible and enjoyable, encouraging you to continue striving for your wellness goals.

Cultivating a positive mindset and focusing on the intrinsic benefits of yoga can enhance your motivation. Reminding yourself of the physical, mental, and emotional improvements you have experienced through yoga can reinforce your dedication to the practice. Embracing yoga as a lifelong journey of self-improvement and wellness fosters a deep sense of purpose and fulfillment, making it easier to stay motivated and committed to your long-term health and happiness.

8-Week Guide to Senior Health and Fitness through Stretching

Below is a comprehensive table listing 10 essential stretching exercises designed for seniors, tailored for an 8-Week Guide to Senior Health and Fitness through Stretching. Each exercise includes the recommended time allocation to ensure a balanced and effective stretching routine.

Serial Number	Exercise Name	Time Allocated
1.	Seated Neck Stretch	5 minutes
2.	Shoulder Rolls	5 minutes
3.	Seated Cat-Cow Stretch	5 minutes
4.	Seated Forward Bend	5 minutes
5.	Seated Leg Extensions	5 minutes
6.	Ankle Circles	5 minutes
7.	Seated Side Stretch	5 minutes
8.	Seated Marching	5 minutes
9.	Gentle Spinal Twist	5 minutes
10.	Seated Hamstring Stretch	5 minutes

Exercise Descriptions

1. Seated Neck Stretch
   - Description: Gently tilt your head towards each shoulder, holding briefly to stretch the neck muscles.

- Benefits: Relieves tension and improves neck flexibility.

2. Shoulder Rolls
   - Description: Slowly roll your shoulders forward and backward in a circular motion.
   - Benefits: Enhances shoulder mobility and reduces stiffness.

3. Seated Cat-Cow Stretch
   - Description: Alternate between arching your back (cat) and dipping it down (cow) while seated.
   - Benefits: Increases spinal flexibility and alleviates back tension.

4. Seated Forward Bend
   - Description: Slowly bend forward from the hips, reaching towards your feet while keeping your back straight.
   - Benefits: Stretches the lower back and hamstrings, promoting relaxation.

5. Seated Leg Extensions
   - Description: Extend one leg straight out and hold, then lower it back down. Repeat with the other leg.
   - Benefits: Strengthens the quadriceps and improves knee joint flexibility.

6. Ankle Circles
   - Description: Lift one foot off the ground and rotate your ankle clockwise and then counterclockwise. Switch feet.
   - Benefits: Enhances ankle mobility and reduces stiffness.

7. Seated Side Stretch
   - Description: Reach one arm overhead and lean to the opposite side, holding the stretch before switching sides.
   - Benefits: Stretches the oblique muscles and improves lateral flexibility.

8. Seated Marching
   - Description: Lift your knees alternately in a marching motion while seated.
   - Benefits: Promotes circulation and strengthens the hip flexors.

9. Gentle Spinal Twist
   - Description: Rotate your upper body to one side while keeping your hips facing forward. Hold and switch sides.
   - Benefits: Increases spinal mobility and aids in digestion.

10. Seated Hamstring Stretch
   - Description: Extend one leg forward, keeping the knee slightly bent, and reach towards your toes. Hold and switch legs.
   - Benefits: Stretches the hamstrings and lower back, enhancing overall flexibility.

Weekly Structure Overview

- Weeks 1-2: Focus on foundational stretches such as Seated Neck Stretch, Shoulder Rolls, and Seated Marching to build basic flexibility and circulation.
- Weeks 3-4: Introduce Seated Cat-Cow Stretch, Seated Forward Bend, and Seated Leg Extensions to enhance spinal and leg flexibility.
- Weeks 5-6: Incorporate Ankle Circles, Seated Side Stretch, and Gentle Spinal Twist to improve joint mobility and lateral flexibility.
- Weeks 7-8: Combine all exercises with increased hold times and repetitions to solidify gains in strength and flexibility.

Tips for Success

- Consistency: Aim to perform the stretching routine at least 5 days a week.
- Breathing: Focus on deep, steady breaths to maximize relaxation and effectiveness of each stretch.
- Comfort: Use a comfortable chair with back support and ensure you have enough space to move safely.
- Listen to Your Body: Move gently and avoid pushing into any painful positions. Modify exercises as needed to suit your comfort level.

By following this structured 8-week plan, seniors can significantly improve their joint health, flexibility, and overall fitness through safe and effective stretching exercises.

10 Essential Stretching Exercises and Additional Important Activities

In addition to the stretching exercises, it's essential for seniors to incorporate other healthy habits and activities into their daily routines to maximize overall health and fitness. Below are two comprehensive tables: one for the 10 Essential Stretching Exercises and another for Additional Important Activities that complement the stretching routine. Each entry includes the activity name and the recommended time allocation to ensure a balanced and effective 8-week health and fitness program for seniors.

Table 1: Essential Stretching Exercises for Seniors

S/n	Exercise Name	Time Allocated	Description
1.	Seated Neck Stretch	5 minutes	Gently tilt your head towards each shoulder, holding briefly to stretch the neck muscles.
2.	Shoulder Rolls	5 minutes	Slowly roll your shoulders forward and backward in a circular motion.
3.	Seated Cat-Cow Stretch	5 minutes	Alternate between arching your back (cat) and dipping it down (cow) while seated.
4.	Seated Forward Bend	5 minutes	Slowly bend forward from the hips, reaching towards your feet while keeping your back str
5.	Seated Leg Extensions	5 minutes	Extend one leg straight out and hold, then lower it back down. Repeat with the other leg.
6.	Ankle Circles	5 minutes	Lift one foot off the ground and rotate your ankle clockwise and then counterclockwise. Switch feet
7.	Seated Side Stretch	5 minutes	Reach one arm overhead and lean to the opposite side, holding the stretch before switching sides
8.	Seated Marching	5 minutes	Lift your knees alternately in a marching motion while seated.
9.	Gentle Spinal Twist	5 minutes	Rotate your upper body to one side while keeping your hips facing forward. Hold and switch sides

| 10. | Seated Hamstring Stretch | 5 minutes | Extend one leg forward, keeping the knee slightly bent, and reach towards your toes. Hold and switch legs. |

Table 2: Additional Important Activities for Seniors

S/n	Activity Name	Time Allocated	Description
1.	Warm-Up Routine	5 minutes	Begin with gentle movements like shoulder shrugs and arm swings to prepare the body for stretching.
2.	Hydration Breaks	2 minutes	Take short breaks to drink water, ensuring proper hydration throughout the exercise session.
3.	Breathing Exercises	5 minutes	Practice deep, mindful breathing to enhance relaxation and oxygenate the muscles.
4.	Balance Exercises	5 minutes	Incorporate simple balance activities like seated leg lifts or standing near a support to improve stability.
5.	Meditation or Mindfulness	10 minutes	Engage in guided meditation or mindfulness practices to reduce stress and enhance mental well-being.
6.	Cool-Down Routine	5 minutes	Finish with gentle stretches and deep breathing to relax the muscles and lower the heart rate.
7.	Nutritional Planning	10 minutes	Plan balanced meals rich in anti-inflammatory foods to support joint health and overall wellnes
8.	Posture Improvement	Throughout the day	Practice maintaining good posture during daily activities to reduce strain on the joints and muscles

| 9. | Light Strength Training | 10 minutes | Use light weights or resistance bands for exercises like bicep curls and leg presses to build muscle strength. |
| 10. | Sleep Hygiene Practices | Evening routine | Establish a consistent bedtime routine to ensure adequate rest and recovery each night. |

Weekly Structure Overview

- **Weeks 1-2: Foundation Building**

- Stretching Exercises: Focus on foundational stretches such as Seated Neck Stretch, Shoulder Rolls, and Seated Marching.
- Additional Activities: Incorporate warm-up routines, hydration breaks, and basic breathing exercises.

- **Weeks 3-4: Enhancing Flexibility and Balance**

- Stretching Exercises: Add Seated Cat-Cow Stretch, Seated Forward Bend, and Seated Leg Extensions.
- Additional Activities: Introduce balance exercises and begin light strength training.

- **Weeks 5-6: Increasing Mobility and Strength**

- Stretching Exercises: Incorporate Ankle Circles, Seated Side Stretch, and Gentle Spinal Twist.
- Additional Activities: Add meditation sessions and enhance nutritional planning.

- Weeks 7-8: Consolidating Gains and Establishing Routine

- Stretching Exercises: Combine all exercises with increased hold times and repetitions.
- Additional Activities: Focus on cool-down routines, posture improvement, and sleep hygiene practices.

Tips for Success

- Consistency: Aim to perform the stretching and additional activities at least 5 days a week.

- Listening to Your Body: Move gently and avoid pushing into any painful positions. Modify exercises as needed to suit your comfort level.
- Comfort and Safety: Use a comfortable chair with back support, ensure you have enough space to move safely, and keep necessary items (like water) nearby.
- Progress Tracking: Keep a journal to note progress, any discomfort, and how you feel each day to stay motivated and make necessary adjustments.

Integrating both stretching exercises and additional healthy habits into a structured 8-week plan, you can significantly improve their joint health, flexibility, strength, and overall well-being. This comprehensive approach ensures a balanced and sustainable path to enhanced health and fitness.